Oral Medicine and ͏ ͏ogy at a Glance

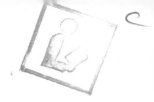

THE SANDE͏
Learning P
C͏ ͏nski

Oral Medicine and Pathology at a Glance

Professor Crispian Scully CBE, MD, PhD, MDS, MRCS, BSc, FDSRCS, FDSRCPS, FFDRCSI, FDSRCSE, FRCPath, FMedSci, FHEA, FUCL, DSc, DChD, DMed(HC), Dr HC

Professor of Oral Medicine, Pathology and Microbiology, University of London; Director (Special Projects) UCL-Eastman Dental Institute; Professor of Special Care Dentistry; Chair of Division of Maxillofacial Diagnostic, Medical and Surgical Sciences
President-elect: International Academy of Oral Oncology (IAOO)
Visiting Professor, Universities of Bristol, Edinburgh and Helsinki

Professor Oslei Paes de Almeida DDS, MSc, PhD

Department of Oral Diagnosis and Pathology, Dental School of Piracicaba, University of Campinas, São Paulo, Brasil

Professor Jose Bagan MD, PhD, MDS

Professor of Oral Medicine. Valencia University, Department of Stomatology, University General Hospital, Valencia, Spain

Professor Pedro Diz Dios MD, DDS, PhD

Senior Lecturer in Special Needs Dentistry
Head of Special Needs Dentistry Section, School of Medicine and Dentistry, Santiago de Compostela University, Spain
Honorary Visiting Professor at UCL-Eastman Dental Institute, University College of London (UK)

Professor Adalberto Mosqueda Taylor DDS, MSc

Professor of Oral Pathology and Medicine,
Health Care Department,
Universidad Autónoma Metropolitana Xochimilco,
Honorary Professor at National Institute of Cancerology,
Mexico, DF

⊛WILEY-BLACKWELL
A John Wiley & Sons, Ltd., Publication

This edition first published 2010
© 2010 Blackwell Publishing Ltd

Blackwell Publishing was acquired by John Wiley & Sons in February 2007. Blackwell's publishing programme has been merged with Wiley's global Scientific, Technical, and Medical business to form Wiley-Blackwell.

Registered office
John Wiley & Sons Ltd, The Atrium, Southern Gate, Chichester, West Sussex, PO19 8SQ, United Kingdom

Editorial offices
9600 Garsington Road, Oxford, OX4 2DQ, United Kingdom
2121 State Avenue, Ames, Iowa 50014-8300, USA

For details of our global editorial offices, for customer services and for information about how to apply for permission to reuse the copyright material in this book please see our website at www.wiley.com/wiley-blackwell.

Library of Congress Cataloging-in-Publication Data

Oral medicine and pathology at a glance / Crispian Scully . . . [et al.].
      p. ; cm. – (At a glance series)
   Includes index.
   ISBN 978-1-4051-9985-8 (pbk. : alk. paper)
   1. Oral medicine–Handbooks, manuals, etc.   2. Mouth–Pathophysiology–Handbooks, manuals, etc.
I. Scully, Crispian.   II. Series: At a glance series (Oxford, England).
   [DNLM: 1. Jaw Diseases–pathology–Handbooks.   2. Mouth Diseases–pathology–Handbooks.
WU 49 O627 2010]
   RC815.O677 2010
   617.5′22–dc22
                                                                    2009037338

A catalogue record for this book is available from the British Library.

Set in 9/11.5pt Times by Graphicraft Limited, Hong Kong
Printed and bound in Singapore by Fabulous Printers Pte Ltd.

1   2010

Contents

Preface

At a Glance books are used by students as introductory texts at the start of a course, or for revision purposes in the run up to examinations. The premise of the series is that the books should cover core information for undergraduates – and this information is broken down into "bite-size chunks". The books will therefore be the foundations for use in practice.

Oral medicine and pathology are subjects which vary across the world in their autonomy, strength, and official recognition, and whose remit varies somewhat from the treatment of oral diseases in ambulatory patients to the care of patients with a wide range of medical and surgical disorders. Oral diseases are seen worldwide, and with increasing global travel and migrations, conditions more common in the tropics are now seen in most countries.

The aim of this book is to offer an overview of aspects of oral medicine and pathology, with an emphasis on oral health care provision in general practice. Intended outcomes are that, having read this book, readers should be more aware of the immediate steps needed to make the diagnosis and arrange patient management.

The authors are specialists and teachers in oral medicine and pathology from two continents, Europe and the Americas, whose focus ranges from mainly in oral medicine to largely in oral pathology, whose experience covers all these conditions and have between them taught in North America, South America, Europe, the Middle East, and the Antipodes. The authors have a common philosophy of recognizing that the mouth is only part of the patient; that prevention and early diagnosis are crucial; that care of the patient is not simply attention to the oral problem; that patients should be empowered in their health care; and that the care is best delivered by a multidisciplinary team, of which oral health care providers are an integral and important part.

The book includes the most important conditions in oral medicine and pathology (those causing pain or affecting the mucosae, salivary glands, or jaws) essential for students – those that are most common and those that are dangerous or even potentially lethal, and is intended to represent current practice at most major centers across the world. The intimate connection with general medicine is highlighted by the various eponymous conditions highlighted in this book. Being restricted by size and cost, this book does not strive to be comprehensive or to include material that is usually covered in courses in Applied Basic Sciences or Human Disease, and does not include diseases of the teeth, or the basics of history taking – only specific relevant points in the text.

Clinicians should bear in mind, however, that the history gives the diagnosis in about 80% of cases. The history is followed by thorough physical examination and often then by investigations, whereupon a diagnosis or at least a differential diagnosis is formulated. Management follows and is usually medical or surgical.

The diagnosis and management is discussed here and, in many cases, practitioners who have the competence can undertake the care; in other cases or if in doubt, it is better that the practitioner refers the patient to a specialist in oral medicine, for an opinion, shared care, or for care by the specialist. Reliable evidence for the effectiveness of many treatment regimens is becoming available but data are sparse and there are thus still many gaps in knowledge, especially in relation to many of the newer biological response modifiers.

The material included in this book is all new, but we have drawn on publications by the authors, especially from Scully C (2008) *Oral and Maxillofacial Medicine* 2nd edition, Churchill Livingstone, Edinburgh, Scully C, Flint SF, Porter SR, Moos K (2004) *Atlas of Oral and Maxillofacial Diseases* 3rd edition, Taylor and Francis, London, and Brown J and Scully C (2004) Advances in oral health care imaging. *Private Dentistry*, **9**, 1, 86–90; **2**, 67–71 and **3**, 78–79.

We thank our patients and also thank Dr Derren Ready (UCL) for microbiology images, and Dr Jane Luker (Bristol) for checking our advice on modern imaging.

Crispian Scully
Oslci Paes de Almeida
Jose Vicente Bagan
Pedro Diz Dios
Adalberto Mosqueda Taylor

"What one knows, one sees"
Goethe (1749–1832)

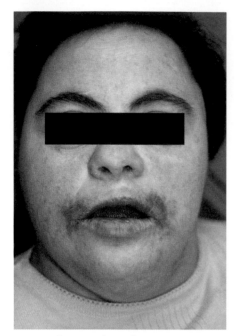

Figure 1.1 Down syndrome facies.

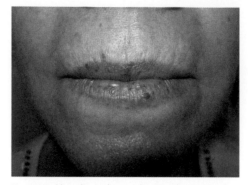

Figure 1.2 Hereditary hemorrhagic telangiectasia.

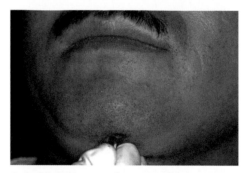

Figure 1.3 Cutaneous odontogenic fistula.

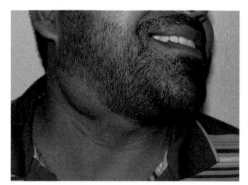

Figure 1.4a Lipoma.

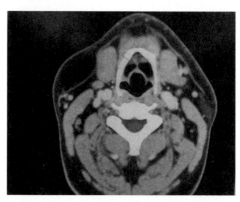

Figure 1.4b Scan of lipoma.

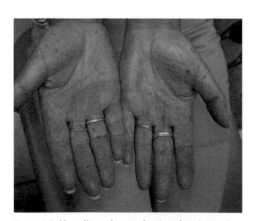

Figure 1.5 Hereditary hemorrhagic telangiectasia (same patient as in Figure 1.2).

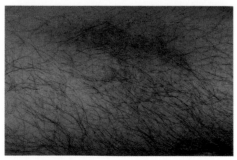

Figure 1.6 Purpura on arm.

This book does not include the basics of history taking, only specific relevant points in the text. *Bear in mind that the history gives the diagnosis in about 80% of cases.*

Following the history, during which the clinician will note the patient's conscious level, any anxiety, appearance, communication, posture, breathing, movements, behavior, sweating, weight loss or wasting (Figure 1.1), physical examination is indicated. This necessitates touching the patient; therefore, informed consent and confidentiality are required, a chaperone available, and religious and cultural aspects should be borne in mind (see Scully and Wilson).

Relevant medical problems may even be manifest in the fully clothed patient – where changes affect the head and neck, cranial nerves, or limbs. Therefore, while there is no rigid system for examination, the clinician should ensure that these areas are checked.

Head and neck

Pupil size should be noted (e.g. dilated in anxiety or cocaine abuse, constricted in heroin abuse).

Facial color should be noted:
- pallor (e.g. anemia)
- rashes (e.g. viral infections, lupus) (Figure 1.2)
- erythema (e.g. anxiety, alcoholism, polycythemia)
  Swellings, sinuses or fistulas should be noted (Figure 1.3).

Facial symmetry is examined for evidence of enlarged masseter muscles (masseteric hypertrophy) suggestive of clenching or bruxism.

Neck swellings should be elicited, followed by careful palpation of lymph nodes (and salivary and thyroid glands), searching for swelling and/or tenderness, by observing the patient from in front, noting any obvious asymmetry or swelling (Figure 1.4a and b), then standing behind the seated patient to palpate the nodes. Systematically, each region needs to be examined lightly with the pulps of the fingers, trying to roll the nodes against harder underlying structures.

Some information can be gained by the texture and nature of the lymphadenopathy; nodes that are tender may be inflammatory (lymphadenitis), while those that are increasing in size and are hard, or fixed to adjacent tissues, may be malignant.

Cranial nerves

The cranial nerves should be examined, in particular facial movement and corneal reflex should be tested and facial sensation determined (Table 1.1). Movement of the mouth as the patient speaks is important, especially when they allow themselves the luxury of some emotional expression.

Facial movement is tested out by asking the patient to:
- close their eyes; any palsy may become obvious, with the affected eyelid failing to close and the globe turning up so that only the white of the eye shows (Bell sign)
- close their eyes tightly against your attempts to open them, and note the degree of force required to part the eyelids
- wrinkle their forehead, and check any difference between the two sides
- smile
- bare the teeth or purse the lips
- blow out the cheeks
- whistle

The muscles of the upper face (around the eyes and forehead) are bilaterally innervated and thus loss of wrinkles on one-half of the forehead or absence of blinking suggests a lesion in the lower motor neurone.

Corneal reflex depends on the integrity both of the trigeminal and facial nerves – a defect of either will give a negative response. This is tested by gently touching the cornea with a wisp of cotton wool twisted to a point. Normally, this procedure causes a blink but, provided that the patient does not actually see the cotton wool, no blink follows if the cornea is anesthetic from a lesion involving the ophthalmic division of the trigeminal nerve, or if there is facial palsy.

Facial sensation is tested by determining the response to light touch (cotton wool) and pin–prick (gently pricking the skin with a sterile pin, probe or needle without drawing blood). It is important to test sensation in all parts of the facial skin but the most common defect is numb chin, due to a lesion affecting the mandibular division of the trigeminal.

Occasionally, a patient complains of hemifacial or complete facial hypoesthesia (reduced sensation) or anesthesia (complete loss of sensation). If the corneal reflex is retained or there is apparent anesthesia over the angle of the mandible (an area not innervated by the trigeminal nerve), then the symptoms are probably functional (non-organic, i.e. psychogenic).

Limbs

Hands may reveal rashes (Figure 1.5), purpura (Figure 1.6), pigmentation or conditions such as arthritis and Raynaud phenomenon. Finger clubbing may reveal systemic disease. Nail changes may reveal anxiety (nail biting), or disease such as koilonychia (spoon-shaped nails), in iron deficiency.

The operator should then ensure that all relevant oral areas are examined, in a systematic fashion.

Reference

Scully C and Wilson N (2006). *Culturally Sensitive Oral Healthcare.* Quintessence, London.

Table 1.1 Cranial nerve examination.

Cranial nerve		Examination
I	Olfactory	Sense of smell for common odors
II	Optic	Visual acuity (Snellen types ⊥ ophthalmoscopy); nystagmus
		Visual fields (by confrontation)
		Pupil responses to light and accommodation
III	Oculomotor	Eye movements
		Pupil responses
IV	Trochlear	Eye movements
V	Trigeminal	Sensation over face ± corneal reflex ± taste sensation
		Motor power of masticatory muscles; jaw jerk
VI	Abducens	Eye movements
VII	Facial	Motor power of facial muscles
		Corneal reflex ± taste sensation
VIII	Vestibulocochlear	Hearing (tuning fork at 256 Hz)
		Balance
IX	Glossopharyngeal	Gag reflex
		Taste sensation
X	Vagus	Gag reflex
XI	Accessory	Motor power of trapezius and sternomastoid
XII	Hypoglossal	Motor power of tongue

2 Examination of mouth, jaws, temporomandibular region and salivary glands

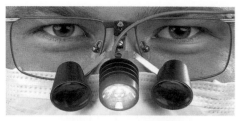

Figure 2.1a Portable miniature operative light.

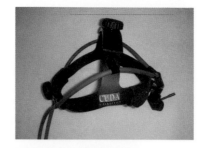

Figure 2.1b ENT headlight.

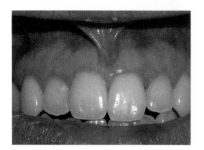

Figure 2.2a Teeth and gingivae.

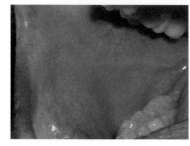

Figure 2.2b Buccal mucosa.

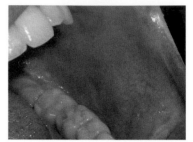

Figure 2.2c Buccal mucosa.

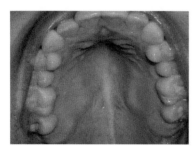

Figure 2.2d Palate.

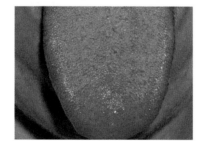

Figure 2.2e Tongue dorsum.

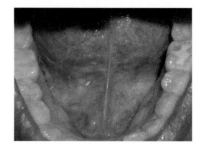

Figure 2.2f Tongue ventrum and floor of mouth.

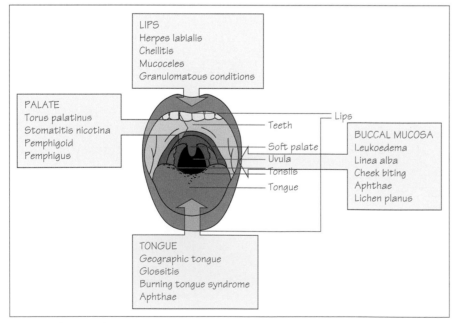

Figure 2.3 Common diseases.

LIPS
Herpes labialis
Cheilitis
Mucoceles
Granulomatous conditions

PALATE
Torus palatinus
Stomatitis nicotina
Pemphigoid
Pemphigus

Teeth
Lips
Soft palate
Uvula
Tonsils
Tongue

BUCCAL MUCOSA
Leukoedema
Linea alba
Cheek biting
Aphthae
Lichen planus

TONGUE
Geographic tongue
Glossitis
Burning tongue syndrome
Aphthae

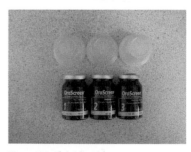

Figure 2.4 Toluidine blue.

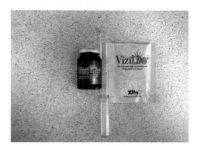

Figure 2.5 Chemiluminescent illumination system (ViziLite).

The lips are best first inspected. Complete visualization intraorally requires a good light; this can be a conventional dental unit light, or special loupes or ENT light (Figures 2.1a and b). If the patient wears a dental appliance, this should be removed to examine beneath.

Mouth

The dentition and occlusion should be examined. Study models on a semi- or fully-adjustable articulator may be needed. This is discussed in basic dental textbooks.

All mucosae should be examined, beginning away from the focus of complaint or location of known lesions. Labial, buccal, floor of the mouth, ventrum of tongue, dorsal surface of tongue, hard and soft palate mucosae, gingivae and teeth should be examined in sequence, recording lesions on a diagram (Figures 2.2a–f). Lesions are described as in Table 2.1.

Some conditions are found only in, or typically in, certain sites (Figure 2.3).

Mucosal lesions are not always readily visualized and, among attempts to aid this, are:
• toluidine blue (vital) staining
• chemiluminescent illumination
• fluorescence spectroscopy and imaging

Toluidine blue staining (Figure 2.4) stains mainly pathological areas blue. The patient rinses for 20 seconds with 1% acetic acid to clean the area; then 20 seconds with plain water; then 60 seconds with 1% aqueous toluidine blue solution; then again 20 seconds with a 1% acetic acid; and finally with water for 20 seconds.

Chemiluminescent illumination relies on fluorophores that naturally occur in cells after rinsing the mouth with 1% acetic acid (Figure 2.5) using excitation with a suitable wavelength.

Fluorescence spectroscopy is where tissues are illuminated with light, and lesions change the fluorophore concentration and light scattering and absorption, and their visibility may thus be enhanced.

Jaws

Jaw deformities or lumps may be best confirmed by inspection from above (maxillae/zygomas) or behind (mandible), then palpated to detect swelling or tenderness. The maxillary sinuses can be examined by palpation for tenderness. X-ray (Waters projection), computed tomography (CT), magnetic resonance imaging (MRI), transillumination or endoscopy can help.

Temporomandibular joint (TMJ)

Check:
• opening and closing paths
• opening extent (inter-incisal distance at maximum mouth opening)
• excursions
• joint noises
• condyles, by palpating them with a finger, via the external auditory meatus
• masticatory muscles on both sides; masseters, by intraoral–extraoral compression between finger and thumb, palpate the masseter bimanually by placing a finger of one hand intraorally and the index and middle fingers of the other hand on the cheek over the masseter; note any hypertrophy.

Temporalis: Check by direct palpation of the temporal region. Palpate the temporal origin along the anterior border of the ascending mandibular ramus, asking the patient to clench their teeth.

Lateral pterygoid (lower head): Check by placing a little finger up behind the maxillary tuberosity (the "pterygoid sign"). Examine the muscle indirectly by asking the patient to open the jaw against resistance and to move the jaw to one side while applying gentle resistance.

Medial pterygoid: Check intraorally lingually to the mandibular ramus.

Salivary glands

Oral dryness (scarce or frothy saliva; absence of saliva pool in floor of mouth, reduced flow from Stensen duct, food residues; lipstick on teeth; mirror sticks to mucosa) should be excluded. Salivary function assessment is discussed in Chapter 40.

Major salivary glands (parotids and submandibulars) should be inspected and palpated for evidence of enlargement:
• Parotids are palpated using fingers placed over the glands in front of the ears, to detect pain or swelling. Early enlargement of the parotid gland is characterized by outward deflection of the lower part of the ear lobe, which is best observed by looking at the patient from behind.
• Submandibulars are palpated bimanually between fingers inside the mouth and extraorally.

Table 2.1 Main descriptive terms applied to orofacial and skin lesions.

Term	Meaning
Atrophy	Reduction in tissue mass
Bulla	Visible fluid accumulation within or beneath epithelium (blister)
Cicatrix	Scar: A permanent mark after healing
Cyst	Closed cavity (epithelial lining)
Desquamation	Loss of superficial epithelial thickness (commonly follows a blister)
Ecchymosis	Macular area of hemorrhage > 2 cm in diameter (i.e. a bruise)
Erosion	Loss of most of epithelial thickness (often follows a blister)
Erythema	Redness of mucosa (from atrophy, inflammation, vascular congestion or increased perfusion)
Exfoliation	Splitting off of epithelial keratin in scales or sheets
Fibrosis	Formation of excessive fibrous tissue
Fissure	Linear gap or slit
Fistula	Abnormal connection, lined by epithelium between two epithelium lined organs
Furuncle	Skin pustule or abscess
Gangrene	Death of tissue
Hematoma	Localized collection of blood
Keloid	Heaped-up scar
Macule	Circumscribed alteration in color or texture, not raised
Nevus	A colored lesion present from birth
Nodule	Solid mass under/within mucosa or skin > 0.5 cm in diameter
Papule	Circumscribed palpable elevation < 0.5 cm in diameter
Petechia	Punctate hemorrhagic spot 1–2 mm in diameter
Plaque	Elevated area of mucosa or skin > 0.5 cm in diameter
Pustule	Visible accumulation of pus in epithelium
Scar	Fibrous tissue replacement of another tissue
Sclerosis	Induration of submucosal and/or subcutaneous tissues
Sinus	A pouch or cavity in any organ or tissue
Tumor	Swelling caused by normal or pathological material or cells
Ulcer	Loss of epithelium with loss of some underlying tissues
Urticaria*	Area of edema, compressible and usually evanescent
Vesicle	Small (< 0.5 cm) visible fluid accumulation in epithelium
Weal*	Area of edema, compressible and usually evanescent

*same

Investigations: Histopathology

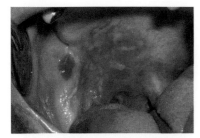

Figure 3.1a Pemphigoid.

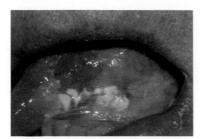

Figure 3.1b Erythroleukoplakia.

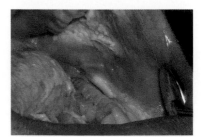

Figure 3.1c White sponge nevus.

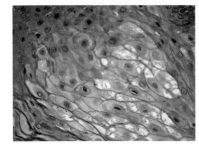

Figure 3.1d White sponge nevus. Typical perinuclear halo 40 ×.

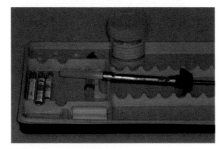

Figure 3.2 Biopsy kit.

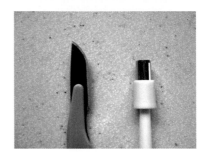

Figure 3.3 Scalpel and punch.

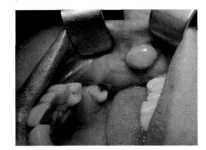

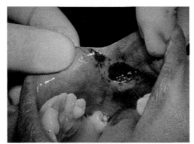

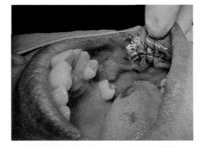

Figure 3.4 Excision biopsy of a lump.

Table 3.1 Biopsy of oral lesions.

Type of lesion	Biopsy	Lesional area to biopsy	Preferred method
Blister	Incisional	Margin/perilesional or whole blister	Scalpel
Carcinoma (suspected)		Margin	
Erosion		Margin/perilesional	
Erythroplakia		Lesion	Punch or scalpel
Granulomatous		Deep	
Leukoplakia		Any red area	
Lichenoid		Lesion	
Lump (mucosal)	Excisional		Scalpel
Mucocele	Excisional		
Pigmented	Excisional		
Salivary major gland swelling	FNAC or FNAB		US guidance
Salivary minor gland swelling	Palate – incisional Lip – excisional	Labial gland biopsy for xerostomia diagnosis – incisional	Scalpel
Ulcer	Incisional	Margin/perilesional	Scalpel

Box 3.1 Indications for biopsy

Indications for biopsy include lesions that:
- have neoplastic or potentially malignant features
- are enlarging
- persist > 3 weeks
- are of uncertain etiology
- fail to respond to treatment
- cause concern.

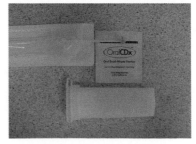

Figure 3.5 Brush biopsy (oral CDx).

Having taken a careful history and completed the clinical examination, the clinician is often in a position to formulate the diagnosis, or at least a list of differential diagnoses. In the latter case, the diagnosis is provisional, and another opinion (e.g. specialist referral) or investigations may be necessary to reach a firm diagnosis.

Informed consent and confidentiality is required for all investigations.

Biopsy is the removal of tissue usually for diagnosis by histopathological examination (Box 3.1). Practitioners who have the competence and confidence can undertake mucosal biopsy but in other cases it may be better to refer.

Methods for biopsy include (Table 3.1):
- *Incisional biopsy* – sampling using a disposable tissue punch (a round-shaped knife) or scalpel. Punches are light, easy to use and less likely than a scalpel to damage anyone. Most biopsies can be performed with a 3 or 5 mm punch, without suturing.
- *Excisional biopsy* – scalpel or laser removal of the whole lesion.
- *Needle biopsy* (mainly for lymph nodes and lumps):
  — **f**ine-**n**eedle **c**utting **b**iopsy (FNCB) using wide-bore needle
  — **f**ine-**n**eedle **a**spiration **b**iopsy (FNA or FNAB) or **c**ytology (FNAC), using 22 gauge needle, sometimes as **u**ltrasound-guided fine-needle aspiration cytology (US-FNAC).
  — curettage; scraping (e.g. from a bone cavity).

Mucosal biopsy

In most incisional biopsies it is preferrable to sample the lesional margin or perilesional area, as sampling an ulcer is rarely helpful since the epithelium has been lost. In suspected malignant mucosal lesions it can be difficult to decide which is the best part to biopsy but, generally, red areas (erythroplakia) are where dysplasia is most likely and therefore are best sampled (Figures 3.1a–d). It can be helpful to stain the mucosa before biopsy with toluidine blue:
- Give a local analgesic (Figure 3.2).
- Use a scalpel when a bullous disorder is suspected as a punch might tear the fragile tissue (Figure 3.3).
- Hold the tissue with suture or forceps to avoid squeezing and causing crush artifacts.

- Remove the required tissue.
- Snap-freeze specimen in liquid nitrogen or place in Michel solution if for immunostaining; if for other staining, place it in 10% neutral buffered formalin (Table 3.2).
- Label specimen and request form carefully and follow the postal regulations if the specimen is to be mailed.
- Suture if necessary, using a fine needle and resorbable suture (e.g. Polyglycolic acid suture (Vicryl* Rapide)), or black silk (Figure 3.4).

Direct immunofluorescence is a qualitative technique used to detect immune deposits (antibodies and/or complement) in the tissues, using fluorescein stain which fluoresces apple green under ultraviolet light, and is useful in the diagnosis, particularly of bullous disorders.

Indirect immunofluorescence is a qualitative and quantitative technique used to detect immune components (circulating antibodies and/or complement) in the serum. It is a two or more stage technique requiring patient serum and animal tissue.

Other techniques

Immunohistochemistry, polymerase chain reaction (PCR) *in situ* hybridization (ISH), and fluorescent ISH (FISH) are also used, especially in diagnosis of infections or neoplasms.

Brush biopsy

This uses a cytobrush as a sampling device to reach deeper layers of the oral epithelium (Figure 3.5), evaluating the cells obtained by computer-assisted image analysis. Major limitations are cost and high false-negative rates.

Labial salivary gland biopsy

- Give local analgesia.
- Make a linear mucosal incision to one side of the midline in the lower labial mucosa or an X-shaped incision over the swelling which overlies the salivary gland.
- Excise at least four lobules of salivary gland.
- Suture the wound if necessary.

Table 3.2 Frequently used tissue stains.

Stain	Constituents	Stains	Used for
Congo red	Sodium salt of benzidine diazo	Amyloid apple-green under polarized light	Diagnosis of amyloidosis
H&E	Hematoxylin (basic stain)	Cell nuclei (basophilic) stain blue/purple	Most histopathology
	Eosin (acidic stain)	Cytoplasm, connective tissue and other extracellular substances (eosinophilic) stain pink/red	
Mucicarmine	Carmine and aluminium hydroxide	Acid mucins stain pink	Muco-epidermoid carcinoma, Cryptococcus
Papanicolaou (Pap) staining	Combination of hematoxylin, eosin Y, Orange G, Light Green SF and Bismark brown	Nuclei stain blue, cytoplasm of basal cells light blue, intermediate cells orange-red and superficial yellow	Smears for cytopathology
PAS	Periodic acid Schiff	Carbohydrates stain purple	Fungal hyphae, glycogen, mucus
Prussian blue	Potassium ferrocyanide and acid	Iron stains blue or purple	Iron in bone marrow and other biopsy specimens
Romanowsky stains (Wright, Jenner, Leishman, Giemsa)	Eosin Y, methylene blue (methanol and glycerol)	Leukocytes stain purple	Inspection of blood cells
Silver staining	Silver nitrate	Proteins and DNA stain brown/black	Fungi, some bacteria (syphilis, rhinoscleroma), collagen, reticulin
Sudan stains	Sudan III, IV and Black B, Oil Red O	Lipids stain black or red	Lipid deposits
Van Gieson stain	Picric acid and acid fuchsin	Collagen stains red	Collagen in vessels, liver and bone marrow
		Muscle stains yellow	
		Nuclei stain black	

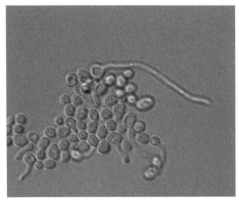

Figure 4.1a *Unstained Candida albicans.*

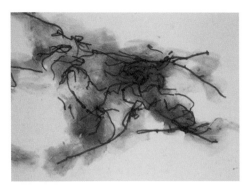

Figure 4.1b *Candida* hyphae PAS staining.

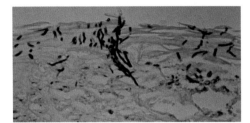

Figure 4.1c *Candidosis* (silver stain).

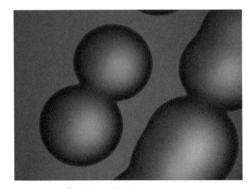

Figure 4.1d *Candida colonies.*

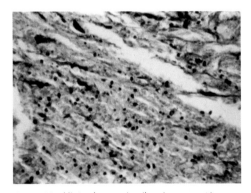

Figure 4.1e *Histoplasmosis silver impregnation.*

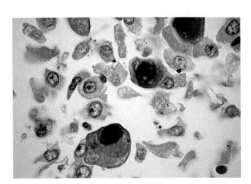

Figure 4.1f *CMV immunohistochemistry.*

Table 4.1 Common microbiological stains.

Stain	Main components	Main uses
Acid fast (Ziehl-Neelsen and Kinyoun stains)	Carbol fuchsin and methylene blue	Differentiates bacteria with waxy cell walls, e.g. *Mycobacterium tuberculosis*, *Mycobacterium leprae*, and *Mycobacterium avium-intracellulare* complex from those that do not
Gomori methenamine silver (GMS)	Silver	Stains carbohydrates in fungi
Gram	Crystal violet, Gram's iodine and safranin	Stains Gram-positive bacteria (e.g. *Staphylococci*), and Gram-negative bacteria (e.g. *Escherichia coli*) based on differences in cell wall structure
Periodic acid Schiff (PAS)	Periodic acid selectively oxidizes glucose, creating aldehydes that react with Schiff to produce a purple-magenta colour	Stains carbohydrates in fungi

Informed consent and confidentiality is required for all investigations.

Testing for infections can be a very sensitive issue, especially in the case of Human Immunodeficiency Virus (HIV) infections, tuberculosis and sexually transmitted infections (e.g. Syphilis, Herpes, Anogenital warts, Gonorrhea). HIV testing in particular remains voluntary and confidential, and patients must be counseled properly beforehand. It has been recommended in the UK that patients should be offered and encouraged to accept HIV testing in a wider range of settings than is currently the case; that patients with specific indicator conditions should be routinely recommended to have an HIV test; and that all doctors, nurses and midwives should be able to obtain informed consent for an HIV test in the same way that they currently do for any other medical investigation (The British HIV Association; British Association of Sexual Health and HIV; and British Infection Society).

Microbiological diagnosis is based on either demonstration of the micro-organism or its components (antigens or nucleic acids), or on the demonstration in the serum of a specific antibody response.

Whenever an early diagnosis is important for the institution of therapy or some other measure (e.g. infection control), methods that demonstrate the organism or its components are best used as results are more speedily obtained.

Micro-organisms can be demonstrated directly in samples or tissues by microscopy using various stains (Table 4.1).

Direct cytological smears and histopathology are sometimes used, as is growth after inoculation in cultures (Figures 4.1a–f), but rapid and sensitive techniques for detecting antigens and nucleic acids have very

much come to the fore (Table 4.2). Antigen tests use, for example, ELISA (Enzyme-Linked ImmunoSorbent Assay), latex agglutination, or immunofluorescence. Nucleic acids are usually detected by polymerase chain reaction (PCR) or variants on that technology.

Microbial specimen handling is important to ensure reliable results. Specimens should be collected before antimicrobials are started and always handled and labelled as a biohazard. If pus is present, a sample should be sent in a sterile container, in preference to a swab. If tuberculosis is suspected, this must be clearly indicated on the request form. If the microbiological specimen cannot be dealt with within two hours, the swab should be placed in transport medium and kept in the refrigerator at 4°C (not a freezer) until dealt with by the microbiology department. Swabs for viral infections must be sent in viral transport medium; dry swabs are no use. Acute and convalescent serum samples should be taken for serological diagnosis of infections. The convalescent serum is collected 2–3 weeks after the acute illness.

Laboratory tests available to help the diagnosis of oral diseases are shown in Table 4.2, but many infections are diagnosed provisionally on clinical grounds. Laboratory confirmation may help diagnosis and management and, in the case of HIV, syphilis and tuberculosis is mandatory.

Reference

The British HIV Association; British Association of Sexual Health and HIV; and British Infection Society. http://www.bhiva.org/files/file1031097.pdf. Accessed 24 March 2009.

Table 4.2 Laboratory diagnostic tests for oral microbial infections*.

Micro-organism	Diagnostic tests		
	Main	Other tests	
Candidosis	Culture in Saboraud dextrose agar for identification	Speciation tests such as germ tube tests and culture on CROM agar	API kits give more definitive identification
Coxsackie	Coxsackie IgM		
Cytomegalovirus (CMV; HHV-5)	CMV IgM	Immunostaining (Figure 4.1f)	
Epstein-Barr virus (EBV)	EBNA IgG	Monospot (Paul-Bunnell heterophile antibody test) is 98% sensitive False negatives common in patients < 5 years (when anti-VCA IgM should be assayed)	
Herpes simplex viruses (HSV)	Immunofluorescence testing (IF) and enzyme linked immunosorbent assays (ELISA), Immunostaining will give same day results Nucleic acid (PCR)	Mouth washing for culture Scrapings of lesions reveal HSV by EM and multinucleate giant Tzanc cells	Serology: HSV IgG and IgM in primary infection HSV specific IgG alone in reactivation Western blot is confirmatory
Herpes varicella-zoster virus (VZV)	Immunostaining Nucleic acid (PCR)	Scrapings of lesions reveal VZV by EM and multinucleate giant Tzanc cells	Serology: VZV IgM in primary and recurrent infections
Mumps	Mumps IgM	Serum amylase raised	Mumps IgG later
Syphilis	Serology Non-specific Reagin tests (VDRL and RPR tests) Specific tests for treponemal antibodies (TPI, FTA-Abs, hemagglutination tests (HATTS and MHA-TP))	Fluorescent antibody staining of smear	Dark ground microscopy
Tuberculosis	Fluorescence staining (auramine-rhodamine) or Ziehl-Neelsen staining or nucleic acid probes	Nucleic acid amplification tests (NAAT) PCR to detect TB DNA Interferon-γ (interferon-gamma) release assays (IGRAs)	Culture MB/BacT, BACTEC 9000, and the Mycobacterial Growth Indicator Tube (MGIT) ELISA Adenosine deaminase

* See Chapter 60 for HIV-testing.

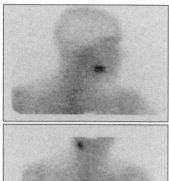
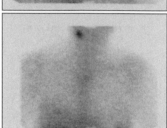

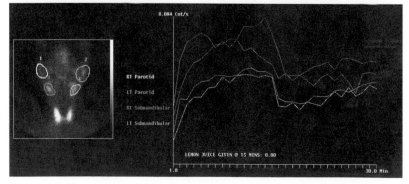

Figure 5.1 Bone Scan: Mandibular squamous cell carcinoma.

Figure 5.3 Gorlin-Goltz syndrome: keratocystic odontogenic tumor.

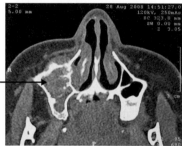

Figure 5.2a CT: osteosarcoma.

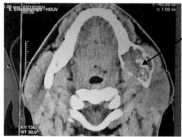
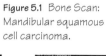

Figure 5.2b CT: ameloblastoma.

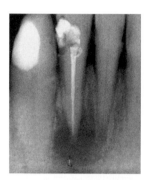

Figure 5.4 Periapical radiography: periapical granuloma.

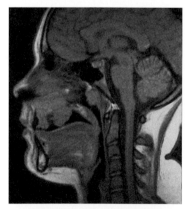

Figure 5.5 MRI: head and neck.

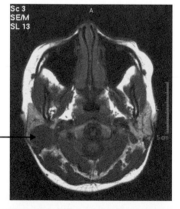

Figure 5.6 MRI: pleomorphic adenoma T1.

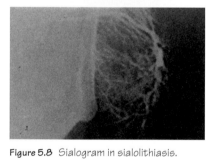

Figure 5.8 Sialogram in sialolithiasis.

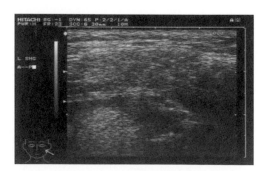

Figure 5.7 Salivary scintiscan normal.

Figure 5.9 Ultrasound scan. Submandibular salivary gland. Courtesy of J. Brown, C. Scully and Private Dentistry.

Informed consent and confidentiality is required for all investigations.

Because of the adverse effects of ionising radiation and the cumulative effect of radiation hazard, clinicians requesting examination or investigation using X-rays must satisfy themselves that each investigation is necessary and that the benefit outweighs the risk.

Ultrasound and magnetic resonance imaging avoid radiation hazards.

Angiography is a relatively high radiation dose invasive technique and MRI angiography is often used in its place. Angiography use should first be discussed with a radiologist, but it can be useful in diagnosis of:
• vascular anomalies or tumors
• parotid gland deep lobe tumors

Arthrography has been used in the past for diagnosis of suspected TMJ internal derangements but, in most centres, it has been superceded by MRI.

Bone scintiscanning is a high radiation dose technique and often other imaging modalities can be more appropriately used. It is essential to discuss with a radiologist prior to referring the patient, but it can be useful in diagnosis of:
• bone invasion or metastases (Figure 5.1)
• condylar or coronoid hyperplasia
• fibro-osseous disease
• other bone disease

Computed axial tomography (CT or CAT) shows the bone and teeth white, and can be useful in diagnosis of:
• hard tissue lesions (Figures 5.2a and b)
• paranasal sinuses diseases
• lesions in complex anatomical areas inaccessible to conventional radiographs
• tumor spread, to exclude cranial base or intracranial pathology
• TMJ disorders (Cone Beam Computed Tomography (CBCT) is especially helpful)

Disadvantages of CT are mainly that it:
• gives a fairly high radiation exposure (CT of the head can give the equivalent exposure to about 100 chest radiographs)
• is expensive
• gives artfacts (star artfacts) when imaging the jaws if amalgam, other metal restorations or implants are present

Cone beam CT is becoming widely utilised for imaging bone/dental pathology of the jaws but is not recommended for imaging soft tissue lesions. It has the advantage of a lower radiation dose to the patient than conventional CT.

Dental panoramic tomography (DPT; or orthopantomography [OPTG]) is a specialized tomographic technique used to produce a flat representation of both jaws, offering a good overview of the dentition, maxillary sinuses, mandibular ramus and temporomandibular joints. It can demonstrate jaw lesions (Figure 5.3) and generalized pathology such as periodontitis, but is subject to considerable and unpredictable geometric distortion, is greatly affected by positioning errors and has relatively low spatial resolution compared with intraoral radiographs. DPT also:
• lacks the detail obtained by intraoral radiography such as periapical films
• does not show caries until it is has progressed to dentine
• does not show detail in the anterior jaws, where the spine is superimposed
• always shows ghost shadows
• images only those tissues within the focal trough.

It has no radiation dose saving advantage over full mouth radiographs since a tissue weighting factor for salivary glands has been included in the calculations of effective dose by the International Commission on Radiological Protection (ICRP).

Intraoral radiography, including periapical, bitewing and occlusal projections, is the basic imaging used for dental pathology and has higher spatial resolution which allows detection of small carious lesions and periapical radiolucencies that may not always be detectable with DPT. It can be useful in diagnosis of:
• approximal caries
• other coronal pathology
• tooth root pathology
• periapical pathology (abscess, granuloma, cyst, etc.) (Figure 5.4)
• adjacent bone pathology.

Magnetic resonance imaging (MRI) does not use ionising radiation, the bone shows black, and it gives good images of soft tissues (Figures 5.5 and 5.6) and is the imaging modality of choice to aid in the diagnosis and management of:
• soft tissue lesions, including malignant lesions (e.g. carcinoma, lymphoma) (Figure 5.6)
• temporomandibular joint disease
• trigeminal neuralgia
• idiopathic facial pain
• children and young people (rather than CT).

The disadvantages of MRI are that it is:
• not as good as CT for imaging bone lesions
• liable to produce image artifacts where metal objects are present (dental restorations, orthodontic appliances, metallic foreign bodies, joint prostheses, implants, etc.)
• expensive.

Contraindications to MRI include:
• implanted electric devices (e.g. heart pacemakers, cardiac defibrillators, nerve stimulators, cochlear implants)
• intracranial vascular clips, if these are ferromagnetic
• prosthetic cardiac valves containing metal
• obesity (weight limit on gantry and size of scanner)
• claustrophobia (unless open scanner available)

Salivary scintiscanning is now very rarely used, since ultrasound has become the imaging modality of choice for assessing salivary glands (Figure 5.7). It can help examine all salivary glands simultaneously, and is useful in the diagnosis of salivary:
• ductal obstruction
• aplasia
• neoplasms
• Sjögren's syndrome.

Sialography examines one major gland only (Figure 5.8) but can be useful in diagnosis of:
• salivary duct obstruction
• intermittent salivary swelling
• recurrent salivary infections.

Contraindications:
• allergy to radiocontrast media (e.g. iodides)
• acute salivary infection.

Ultrasound scanning (US) is non-invasive use of 3.5–10 mHz frequency sound waves, and is the first-line imaging modality to use in:
• diagnosis of soft tissue swellings (e.g. lymph nodes, thyroid or salivary glands) (Figure 5.9)
• diagnosis of soft tissue hard inclusions (e.g. calcification, foreign bodies)
• assisting fine needle aspiration biopsy (ultrasound guided FNA or FNAB) as it improves the diagnostic yield.

Doppler ultrasound is also useful for investigating vascularity of lesions. There are no contraindications to ultrasound, but disadvantages are that it:
• is user dependent
• may fail to visualize the deep extent of a lesion

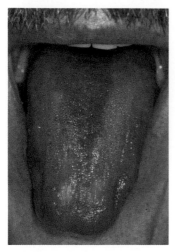

Figure 6.1a Pernicious anemia.

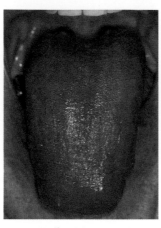

Figure 6.1b Pernicious anemia (resolved after 10 days therapy).

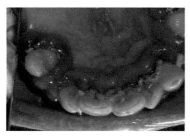

Figure 6.2 Leukemia presenting with gingival lesions.

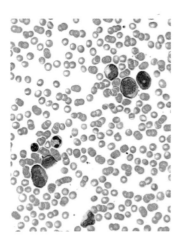

Figure 6.3 Blood film from infectious mononucleosis.

Informed consent and confidentiality is required for all investigations.

Blood contains cells (erythrocytes, leukocytes, platelets), proteins (antibodies, enzymes, etc.) and other substances. Blood tests help determine disease states, but should be the appropriate test and requested only when clinically indicated. Furthermore, abnormal "blood results" do not always mean disease. Apart from technical errors which are possible, some tests assays for autoantibodies, for example (which may be indicated in suspected bullous diseases or Sjögren's syndrome) may show abnormalities (in this case autoantibodies), but these do not always indicate disease and their absence does not necessarily exclude it. There is also a danger of needlestick injury.

Whole blood is used for full blood count (FBC; or full blood picture, FBP) and must be anticoagulated (EDTA in the collection tube). FBP may identify anemia (e.g. in glossitis, burning mouth syndrome, or oral ulceration) (Figures 6.1a and b). The white blood cell count (WBC or WCC) and blood film may reveal leukemia or infection such as infectious mononucleosis (Figures 6.2 and 6.3), and a platelet count can help where bleeding tendency is suspected.

A sickle test should be requested for patients of African heritage (ideally also for those of Mediterranean and Asian origin).

Serum, obtained by collecting whole blood without anticoagulant, is used for assaying antibodies, which can help diagnose infections and autoimmune disorders, and for most biochemical substances (e.g. "liver enzymes").

Table 6.1 shows the interpretation of some blood tests.

Referring a patient for specialist opinion

It is the responsibility of clinicians to recognize the early signs of serious disease and to direct the patient to the appropriate specialist for a second opinion and include any relevant investigation results.

Essential details of a referral letter include:

Name and contact details of the patient
including age, address and day-time telephone number.
Name and contact details of the referring and other clinicians
History of present complaint
brief details and description of the nature and site of lesion(s).
Urgency of referral
Social history
Medical history
Special requirements
e.g. for interpreter, sign language expert or special transport (Scully and Porter, 2007).

Reference

Scully C and Porter SR (2007). Referrals in oral medicine. *Dental Update*, Jul–Aug; **34** (6); 340–342, 345–346, 348–350.

Table 6.1 Interpretation of blood test results[a].

Blood cells	Level ↑[b]	Level ↓[b]
Hemoglobin	Polycythemia	Anemia
Hematocrit (packed cell volume or PCV)	Dehydration	
Mean cell volume (MCV) $MCV = PCV/RBC$	Vitamin B_{12} or folate deficiency, liver disease, alcoholism	Iron deficiency, thalassemia, chronic disease
Mean cell hemoglobin (MCH) $MCH = Hb/RBC$	Pernicious anemia	Iron deficiency, thalassemia
Red cell count (RBC)	Polycythemia	Anemia
Reticulocytes	Hemolytic states	Chemotherapy, bone marrow disease
White cell count (total)	Infection, inflammation, leukemia, trauma, pregnancy	Some infections, bone marrow disease, drugs
Neutrophils	Pregnancy, exercise, infection, trauma, malignancy, leukemia	Some infections, drugs, bone marrow disease
Lymphocytes	Some infections, leukemia, lymphoma	Some infections (e.g. HIV), drugs
Eosinophils	Allergic disease, parasitic infestations	Some immune defects
Platelets	Myeloproliferative disease	Leukemia, drugs, HIV, autoimmune
Biochemistry (on plasma or serum)		
Acid phosphatase	Prostate cancer	—
Alanine transaminase (ALT)	Liver disease, infectious mononucleosis	Hypothyroidism, hypophosphatasia
Albumin	Dehydration	Liver disease, malnutrition, malabsorption, nephrotic syndrome, myeloma
Alkaline phosphatase	Puberty, pregnancy, bone disease	—
Amylase	Pancreatic disease, mumps	—
Angiotensin converting enzyme	Sarcoidosis	—
Aspartate transaminase (AST)	Liver disease, myocardial infarct, trauma	—
Bilirubin (total)	Liver or biliary disease, hemolysis	—
Calcium	Primary hyperparathyroidism, bone tumors, sarcoidosis	Hypoparathyroidism, renal failure, rickets, nephrotic syndrome, chronic renal failure, lack of vitamin D, pancreatitis
Cholesterol	Hypercholesterolemia, pregnancy, hypothyroidism, diabetes, nephrotic syndrome, liver or biliary disease	Malnutrition, hyperthyroidism
Complement (C3)	Trauma; surgery; infection	Liver disease, immune complex diseases, e.g. lupus erythematosus
Complement (C4)	—	Liver disease, immune complex diseases, hereditary angioedema
C1 esterase inhibitor	—	Hereditary angioedema
Erythrocyte sedimentation rate (ESR)	Pregnancy, many diseases	
Ferritin	Liver disease, hemochromatosis, leukemia, lymphoma, thalassemia	Iron deficiency
Folic acid	Folic acid therapy	Alcoholism, dietary deficiency or malabsorption, hemolytic anemias, phenytoin
Free thyroxine index (FTI) (serum T4 and T3 uptake)	Hyperthyroidism	Hypothyroidism
Gammaglutamyl transpeptidase (GGT)	Alcoholism, obesity, liver or renal disease, myocardial infarct	—
Globulins (total) (see also under protein)	Liver disease, multiple myeloma, autoimmune disease, chronic infections	Chronic lymphatic leukemia, malnutrition, protein losing states
Glucose	Diabetes mellitus, pancreatitis, hyperthyroidism, hyperpituitarism, Cushing disease, liver disease	Hypoglycemic drugs, Addison disease, hypopituitarism, liver disease
Total immunoglobulins	Liver disease, infection, sarcoidosis, connective tissue disease	Immunodeficiency, nephrotic syndrome, enteropathy
IgG	Myelomatosis, connective tissue disorders	Immunodeficiency, nephrotic syndrome
IgA	Alcoholic cirrhosis	Immunodeficiency
IgM	Primary biliary cirrhosis, nephrotic syndrome, parasites, infections	Immunodeficiency
IgE	Allergies, parasites	—
Percent carbohydrate-deficient transferrin	Alcoholism	—
Phosphate	Renal failure, bone disease, hypoparathyroidism, hyper-vitaminosis D	Hyperparathyroidism, rickets, malabsorption syndrome
Plasma viscosity	Pregnancy, many diseases	—
Potassium	Renal failure, Addison disease, ACE inhibitors, potassium supplements	Vomiting, diabetes, Conn syndrome, diuretics, Cushing's disease, malabsorption, corticosteroids
Protein (total)	Liver disease, multiple myeloma, sarcoid, connective tissue diseases	Pregnancy, nephrotic syndrome, malnutrition, enteropathy, renal failure, lymphomas
Sodium	Dehydration, Cushing disease	Cardiac failure, renal failure, Addison's disease, diuretics
Steroids (corticosteroids)	Cushing disease, some tumors	Addison's disease, hypopituitarism
Thyroxine (T4)	Hyperthyroidism, pregnancy, oral contraceptive	Hypothyroidism, nephrotic syndrome, phenytoin
Urea	Renal failure, dehydration, gastrointestinal bleed	Liver disease, nephrotic syndrome, pregnancy, malnutrition
Vitamin B_{12}	Liver disease, leukemia, polycythemia rubra vera	Pernicious anemia, gastrectomy, Crohn's disease, vegans

[a] Adults unless otherwise stated. [b] A selection only.

7 Anatomical variants and developmental anomalies

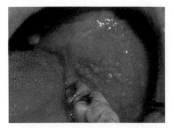
Figure 7.1a Fordyce spots.

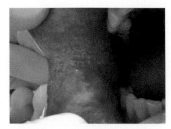
Figure 7.1b Fordyce spots.

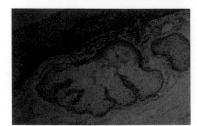
Figure 7.1c Fordyce spots.

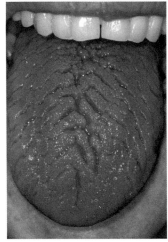
Figure 7.2 Fissured tongue.

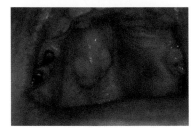
Figure 7.3 Torus palatinus.

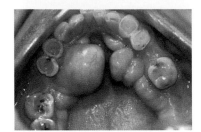
Figure 7.4 Torus mandibularis.

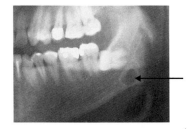
Figure 7.5 Stafne bone cavity.

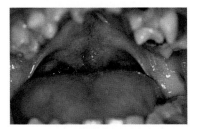
Figure 7.6 Bifid uvula.

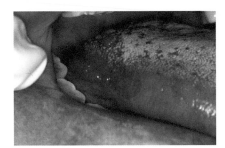
Figure 7.7a Folliate papillitis.

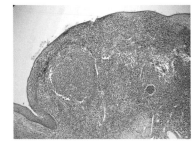
Figure 7.7b Folliate papillitis.

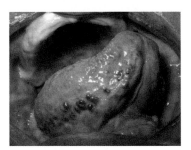
Figure 7.8 Lingual varicosities.

Anatomical features or developmental anomalies that may be noticed by patients and cause concern include:
- Fordyce spots (Figures 7.1a–c)
- fissured tongue (Figure 7.2)
- torus palatinus (Figure 7.3)
- torus mandibularis (Figure 7.4)
- Stafne bone cavity (Figure 7.5)
- unerupted teeth; mainly third molars (Figure 7.5), second premolars, and canines
- pterygoid hamulus; may give rise to concern about an unerupted tooth
- bifid uvula; symptomless (Figure 7.6), but may overlie a submucous cleft palate
- papillae:
  – incisive; may bother the patient if traumatized
  – parotid (orifice of Stensen duct); may occasionally be traumatized by biting or an orthodontic or other appliance
  – lingual foliate; occasionally become inflamed (papillitis) and clinically mimic carcinoma (Figures 7.7a and b)
  – retrocuspid; found on the lingual gingiva in the mandibular canine region, it resembles the incisive papilla
  – leukoedema; a normal variation more prevalent in people who have dark skin, in which there is a white-bluish tinge of the buccal mucosa that disappears when the cheek is stretched
- lingual varicosities (Figure 7.8).

Fordyce spots ("Fordyce granules")

Definition: Small, painless, raised, white or yellowish spots or bumps 1 to 3 mm in diameter seen beneath the buccal or labial mucosa. Similar spots may be seen on genitals (penis or labia).

Prevalence (approximate): Seen in probably 80% of the population.

Age mainly affected: After puberty.

Gender mainly affected: M > F.

Etiopathogenesis: These are sebaceous glands containing neutral lipids similar to those found in skin sebaceous glands, but not associated with hair follicles.

Diagnostic features

History: Often not noticeable until after puberty (although they are present histologically).

Clinical features: Usually seen in the buccal mucosa, particularly inside the commissures, and sometimes in retromolar regions and upper lip. They appear more obvious in males, patients with greasy skin and older people, and they may be increased in some rheumatic disorders.

Differential diagnosis: Thrush or lichen planus. Occasionally they may be mistaken for leukoplakia or Koplik spots (measles).

Diagnosis is clinical: investigations are rarely required.

Management

The spots may become less prominent if isotretinoin is given. CO_2 laser and photodynamic therapy are reportedly effective therapies but no treatment is indicated, only reassurance.

Prognosis

Excellent: They are of cosmetic concern only.

Fissured tongue (scrotal or plicated tongue)

Definition: A tongue with fissures on the dorsum.

Prevalence (approximate): About 5% of population.

Age mainly affected: More noticeable with increasing age.

Gender mainly affected: M = F.

Etiopathogenesis: Hereditary, a fissured tongue is found in many normal persons but is more often seen in psoriasis, Down syndrome (trisomy 21), Job syndrome (hyper-IgE and immunodeficiency) and Melkersson-Rosenthal syndrome (Chapter 27).

Diagnostic features

History: Usually asymptomatic. However, it is often complicated by geographic tongue, or the tongue becomes sore for no apparent reason.

Clinical features: Multiple fissures on the dorsum of the tongue.

Differential diagnosis: Lobulated tongue of Sjögren syndrome or chronic mucocutaneous candidosis.

Diagnosis is clinical: investigations are rarely required. Blood tests are optional if the tongue is sore.

Management

No treatment is indicated or available.

Prognosis

Excellent.

Stafne cyst or bone cavity

This is a lingual, mandibular, focal, bone concavity, classically in the submandibular fossa, below the inferior alveolar canal and close to the mandible inferior margin. Although this radiolucency may appear to be cystic, it is a congenital defect typically measuring less than 2 cm, usually filled with fat but may also contain salivary tissue.

Torus palatinus

Definition: A developmental benign exostosis in the midline of hard palate.

Prevalence (approximate): Up to 20% of the population; seen especially in Asians and Inuits.

Age mainly affected: After puberty.

Gender mainly affected: F > M (2:1).

Etiopathogenesis: Developmental exostosis.

Diagnostic features

History: Symptomless unless ulcerated by trauma.

Clinical features: Most tori occur in the palate, midline and extend symmetrically to either side. Size (most are < 2 cm diameter) and shape (lobular, nodular or irregular) are variable. The lesion is painless, and the surface is bony hard and the overlying mucosa normal and typically of normal color unless traumatized.

Differential diagnosis: Unerupted teeth, cysts or neoplasms.

The diagnosis is usually clinical but radiography may help.

Management

Tori should usually be left alone. Surgery (excision or reduction) is indicated only if causing severe difficulties with dentures.

Prognosis

Excellent.

Torus mandibularis

Definition: Bony lumps usually lingual to mandibular premolars.

Prevalence (approximate): Up to 6%; seen especially in Asians and Inuits.

Age mainly affected: After puberty.

Gender mainly affected: F = M.

Etiopathogenesis: Developmental exostosis but bruxism and parafunction may play a role.

Diagnostic features

Tori are symptomless unless traumatized.

Clinical features: Tori are typically bilateral bony hard lumps, with normal overlying mucosa and typically of normal color or yellowish. They are painless, and the size and shape are variable – but may be lobular, nodular or irregular.

Differential diagnosis: Unerupted teeth, cysts or neoplasms.

The diagnosis is usually clinical but radiography may help.

Management

Tori should usually be left alone. Surgery (excision or reduction) is indicated only if causing severe difficulties with dentures.

Prognosis

Excellent.

Varicosities

Oral varicosities present as purplish blue spots, nodules or ridges, usually asymptomatic, most commonly involving the lingual veins or vessels of the ventral surface of the tongue and the floor of the mouth. Often seen in older people, they are benign and inconsequential. Some cases have been successfully treated with cryosurgery or sclerotherapy.

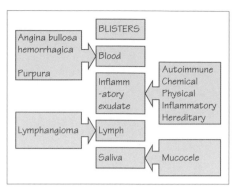

Figure 8.1 Blister causes.

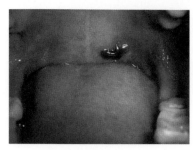

Figure 8.2 Pemphigus simulating angina bullosa hemorrhagica.

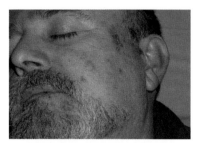

Figure 8.3 Herpes zoster.

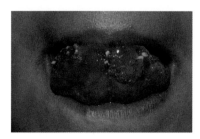

Figure 8.4 Lymphangioma.

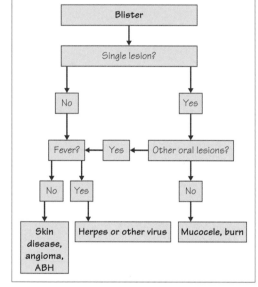

Figure 8.5 Blister diagnosis. ABH-angina bullosa hemorrhagica.

Table 8.1 Main causes of oral blisters.

True blisters	False blisters
Angina bullosa hemorrhagica	Abscesses
Infections	Cysts
Coxsackie and other enteroviruses	**Lymphangiomas**
Herpes simplex virus	**Mucoceles**
Herpes varicella-zoster virus	
Mucocutaneous diseases	
Dermatitis herpetiformis	
Epidermolysis bullosa	
Erythema multiforme	
Lichen planus	
Linear IgA disease	
Pemphigoid	
Pemphigus	
Others	
Amyloidosis	
Burns	
Drugs	
Paraneoplastic disorders	

Table 8.2 Investigations used in oral mucosal disease*.

Procedure	Advantages	Disadvantages	Remarks
Biopsy	Often affords definitive diagnosis	Invasive	Immuno-fluorescence examination is necessary if a bullous disease suspected
Hemoglobin, blood cell count including platelets	Simple, inexpensive	—	Essential in purpura, ulceration, glossitis or angular stomatitis
Serology	Simple, inexpensive and may be diagnostically helpful	Diagnosis of viral infections is delayed or retrospective Autoantibodies may not always mean disease	Essential in suspected autoimmune and other immunological disorders

* See Table 4.2 for microbiological investigations

A vesicle is arbitrarily defined as a blister < 5 mm diameter; a bulla is > 5 mm diameter. Blisters often break down to leave erosions or ulcers and may be seen as a result of a range of causes (Table 8.1). Some other fluid-filled lesions can mimic blistering disorders but in these the lesions usually persist (Figure 8.1).

Burns are a common cause of mouth blistering and may result from hot instruments or hot foods/drinks. Pizza and hot coffee are common culprits. Microwave ovens have been responsible for many oral burns from the very hot food produced; food and drink should never be ingested straight out of the microwave. The diagnosis is usually obvious from the history, and burns in the mouth heal rapidly without intervention unless they are deep.

The most important causes of blistering are the mucocutaneous bullous (skin or vesiculobullous) disorders – pemphigus, pemphigoid, epidermolysis bullosa, erythema multiforme, and some other diseases (Figure 8.2). The bullae are usually filled with clear fluid but those of pemphigoid may sometimes be blood-filled. The bullae may sometimes be induced by rubbing the mucosa or skin (Nikolsky sign). Bullae in the mouth eventually break to leave erosions.

Vesicles and then ulcers may be seen in viral infections, especially in herpes simplex stomatitis, chickenpox, herpangina and hand, foot and mouth disease. Though the immune system eventually eliminates the herpesviruses from most locations, some remain dormant in the sensory ganglia, from which there can be recurrent infections such as herpes labialis, which typically presents at the vesicular stage, or zoster (Figure 8.3), which presents also with pain and rash. The above blisters tend to contain clear fluid.

Superficial mucoceles, caused by extravasation of mucus from minor salivary glands, produce isolated blisters. Mucoceles may be bluish in appearance, especially when in the floor of mouth (ranula). Lymphangiomas may resemble blisters and may be admixed with angiomatous lesions (Figure 8.4). Blood-filled blisters may also be caused by trauma, or by localized oral purpura (angina bullosa hemorrhagica: ABH), rarely by thrombocytopenia, or amyloidosis.

Diagnosis

Blisters in children are most likely to represent burns, viral infections, mucoceles or erythema multiforme. In adults, mucoceles, the skin diseases, ABH and shingles are most common potential causes (Figure 8.5). A useful acronym to remember the causes of blisters is AIM (Angina bullosa hemorrhagica; Infections; Mucocutaneous and mucoceles).

Diagnosis is based on the history and examination but investigations that may well be indicated include blood tests (may be needed to examine for antibodies and confirm hemostasis is normal), and biopsy histopathology and immunostaining for IgG, IgA, or C3 (may be indicated to exclude mucocutaneous diseases) (Table 8.2). Microbiological investigations may be needed if an infectious cause is suspected (Table 4.2).

Management

The underlying cause should be corrected if possible. Treatment with paracetamol for analgesia may be required. Paracetamol (acetaminophen) will also reduce any fever but, if fever is present, a more serious cause is probable and should be excluded. Local antiseptics (aqueous chlorhexidine mouthwashes) may aid resolution and help oral hygiene, which must be maintained by toothbrushing and flossing. It is advisable to use chlorhexidine mouthwash at least one hour after brushing with toothpaste that contains SLS (sodium lauryl sulfate), which can otherwise deactivate the mouthwash. Sucking ice and using topical local anesthetic preparations or benzydamine rinses can help. Ensuring an adequate fluid intake is important, especially in children who can readily become dehydrated. Soft cool foods such as milkshakes, iced tea, and ice cream may be needed. Patients should avoid spicy foods, acidic foods, and foods with sharp edges, like potato chips. Citrus fruits and drinks, and alcohol drinks or mouthwashes are best avoided, as they may cause pain.

This management regimen is also applicable to patients who have oral soreness from other causes.

Angina bullosa hemorrhagica (localized oral purpura; traumatic oral hemophlyctenosis)

Definition: Blood blisters appearing with no defined cause spontaneously or after trivial trauma.

Prevalence (approximate): Uncommon.

Age mainly affected: Older people.

Gender mainly affected: F > M.

Etiopathogenesis: Unclear, though this disorder is analogous to senile purpura, bleeding tendency, autoimmunity or diabetes do not appear to underlie this condition. Corticosteroid inhalers may sometimes predispose.

Diagnostic features

History

Oral: There is rapid onset of blistering over minutes, with breakdown in minutes or hours to a large round ulcer which heals spontaneously.

Extraoral: Occasionally affects the pharynx. Skin lesions are absent.

Clinical features

Oral: Blood blisters are typically solitary, large, and confined to the non-keratinised mucosa – soft palate and occasionally the lateral border of tongue or buccal mucosa.

Extraoral: Pharyngeal blisters may be seen.

Differential diagnosis: Differentiate from pemphigoid and other bullous disorders, trauma, and purpura (due to bleeding disorders or anticoagulant therapy).

Investigations

Blood tests are needed to confirm hemostasis is normal. Biopsy to exclude pemphigoid if that is likely. Immunostaining for IgG, IgA, or C3 consistently are non-contributory.

Management

There is no specific treatment other than reassurance. Most lesions recover spontaneously but airway obstruction has been reported rarely. It may be helpful to burst the blister. Topical analgesics may provide symptomatic relief.

Prognosis

Good.

Blisters, infections: Herpes simplex virus

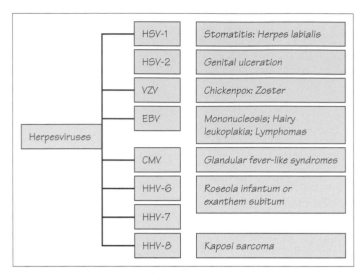

Figure 9.1 Herpesviruses and their diseases.

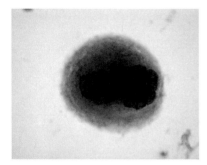

Figure 9.2 HSV pathogenesis.

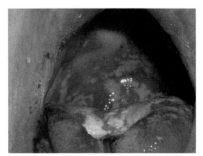

Figure 9.3 Herpetic stomatitis.

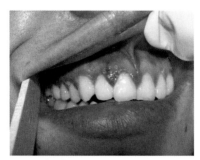

Figure 9.4 Primary herpetic gingivostomatitis.

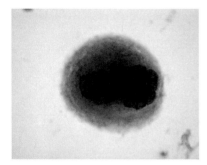

Figure 9.5a Herpes cytology.

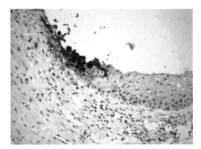

Figure 9.5b Herpes immunostaining.

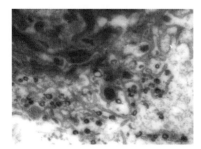

Figure 9.5c Herpes electronmicroscopy.

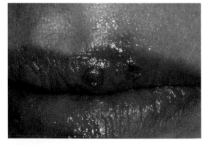

Figure 9.6 Herpes simplex recurrence (herpes labialis).

A range of infections, mainly viral, can produce oral blistering, but most patients present with ulceration after the blisters break. Herpesviruses are frequently responsible (Figure 9.1). Affected patients are largely children and there is often fever, malaise and cervical lymphadenopathy. More severe manifestations and recalcitrant lesions are seen in immunocompromised people.

Herpes simplex

Definition: Herpes simplex virus (HSV) infection is common and affects mainly the mouth (HSV-1 or human herpesvirus-1; HHV-1),

or genitals or anus (HSV-2; HHV-2). Initial oral infection presents as primary herpetic stomatitis (gingivostomatitis). All herpesvirus infections are characterized by latency (Figure 9.2), and can be reactivated. Recurrent disease usually presents as herpes labialis (cold sore).

Prevalence (approximate): Common.

Age mainly affected: Herpetic stomatitis is typically a childhood infection seen between the ages of 2−4 years, but cases are increasingly seen in the mouth and/or pharynx in older patients.

Gender mainly affected: M = F.

Etiopathogenesis: HSV, a DNA virus, is contracted from infected skin, saliva or other body fluids. Most childhood infections are with HSV-1, but HSV-2 is often implicated more often at later ages, often transmitted sexually. UNC-93B1 gene mutations predispose to herpesvirus infection.

Diagnostic features

History: The incubation period is 4–7 days. Some 50% of HSV infections are subclinical and may be thought to be "teething" because of oral soreness.

Clinical features: Primary stomatitis presents with a single episode of multiple oral vesicles which may be widespread, and break down to form ulcers that are initially pinpoint but later fuse to produce irregular painful ulcers (Figure 9.3). Gingival edema, erythema and ulceration are prominent (Figure 9.4). The tongue is often coated and there may be oral malodor.

Herpetic stomatitis probably explains many instances of "teething".

Extraoral features: Commonly include malaise, drooling, fever and cervical lymph node enlargement.

Complications of HSV infection occasionally include erythema multiforme or Bell palsy. HSV-1 appears to increase the risk of developing Alzheimer disease. Rare complications include meningitis, encephalitis and mononeuropathies, particularly in people with impaired immunity, such as infants whose immune responses are still developing, or immunocompromised patients.

Differential diagnosis: Other oral infections and leukemic gingival infiltrates.

Investigations: The diagnosis is largely clinical but blood tests to exclude leukemia (full blood picture and white cell count) may be indicated, and a rising titer of serum antibodies is diagnostically confirmatory but only retrospectively. Cytology, viral DNA sequentiation, culture, immunodetection or electron microscopy are used occasionally (Figures 9.5a–c).

Management

Treatment aims to limit the severity and duration of pain, shorten the duration of the episode, and reduce complications. Management includes a soft diet and adequate fluid intake. Antipyretics/analgesics such as paracetamol help relieve pain and fever. Products containing aspirin must not be given to children with any fever-causing illness suspected of being of viral origin, as this risks causing the serious and potentially fatal Reye syndrome (fatty liver plus encephalopathy). Local antiseptics (0.2% aqueous chlorhexidine mouthwashes) may aid resolution. Aciclovir orally or parenterally is useful especially in immunocompromised patients. Valaciclovir or famciclovir may be needed for aciclovir-resistant infections.

Prognosis

Good, though HSV remains latent thereafter in the trigeminal ganglion and recurrences may occur.

Recurrent herpes labialis

Definition: Recurrent blistering of the lips caused by HSV reactivation.

Prevalence (approximate): ~ 5% of adults.
Age mainly affected: Adults.
Gender mainly affected: M = F.
Etiopathogenesis: HSV latent in the trigeminal ganglion travels to mucocutaneous junctions supplied by the trigeminal nerve, producing lesions on the upper or lower lip, occasionally the nares or the conjunctiva or, occasionally intraoral ulceration. Fever, sunlight, trauma, hormonal changes or immunosuppression can reactivate the virus which is shed into saliva, and there may be clinical recrudescence.

Diagnostic features

History: Oral premonitory symptoms may be tingling or itching sensation on the lip in the day or two days before, followed by appearance of macules, then papules, vesicles and pustules.

Clinical features: Oral lesions start at the mucocutaneous junction and heal usually without scarring in 7–10 days (Figure 9.6). Widespread recalcitrant lesions may appear in immunocompromised patients.

Extraoral: Occasionally lesions become superinfected with *Staphylococcus* or *Streptococcus*, resulting in impetigo. In immunocompromised persons, extensive and persistent lesions may involve the perioral skin. In atopic persons, the lesions of herpes labialis may spread widely to produce eczema herpeticum.

Differential diagnosis: Impetigo and other causes of blisters.

Investigations are rarely needed as the diagnosis is largely clinical.

Management

Penciclovir 1% cream, aciclovir 5% cream or silica gel applied in the prodrome may help abort or control lesions in healthy patients. Systemic aciclovir or other antivirals may be needed for immunocompromised patients.

Prognosis

Usually good but immunocompromised patients can develop recalcitrant lesions.

Recurrent intraoral herpes

Recurrent intraoral herpes in healthy patients tends to affect the hard palate or gingiva, as a small crop of ulcers usually over the greater palatine foramen, following local trauma (e.g. palatal local anesthetic injection), and heals within 1–2 weeks.

Recurrent intraoral herpes in immunocompromised patients may appear as chronic, often dendritic, ulcers frequently on the tongue (herpetic geometric glossitis). Clinical diagnosis tends to underestimate the frequency of these lesions.

Management: The aims are to limit the severity and duration of pain, shorten the duration of the episode, and reduce complications.

Symptomatic treatment with a soft diet and adequate fluid intake, antipyretics/analgesics (paracetamol), local antiseptics (0.2% aqueous chlorhexidine mouthwashes) usually suffices.

Systemic aciclovir or other antivirals may be needed for immunocompromised patients.

Blisters, infections: Varicella zoster virus

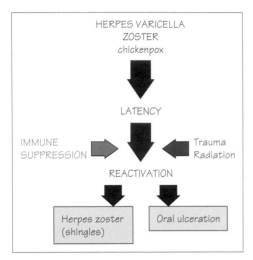

HERPES VARICELLA
ZOSTER
chickenpox

↓

LATENCY

IMMUNE
SUPPRESSION → ↓ ← Trauma
Radiation

REACTIVATION

Herpes zoster
(shingles)   Oral ulceration

Figure 10.1 VZV pathogenesis.

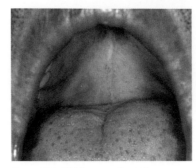

Figure 10.2 Chickenpox ulceration.

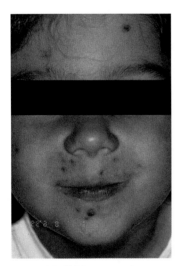

Figure 10.3 Chickenpox rash.

Ophthalmic branch

Maxillary branch

Mandibular branch

Figure 10.4 Trigeminal dermatomes.

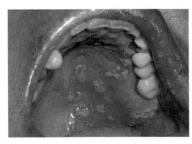

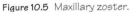

Figure 10.5 Maxillary zoster.

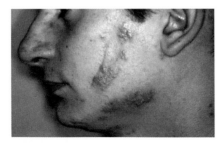

Figure 10.6 Zoster rash.

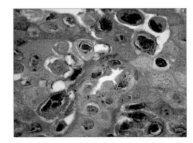

Figure 10.7 Herpes hematoxylin and eosin.

Varicella zoster virus (VZV; human herpesvirus-3; HHV-3) is highly contagious, spreading via droplets from the nasopharynx or contact with secretions. VZV infects the lymphoreticular system, capillary endothelia and epithelia, causing intercellular and intracellular edema and a rash.

The immune system eventually eliminates VZV from most locations and provides lifelong protective immunity from chickenpox, but VZV remains dormant in sensory nerve ganglia (Figure 10.1). Vaccination against VZV will also elicit immunity but further vaccination is necessary five years later.

Chickenpox (varicella)

Definition: A centripetal (concentrated mainly on trunk and head and neck) rash which passes through macular, papular, vesicular and pustular stages.

    Prevalence (approximate): Common.
    Age mainly affected: 4–10 years.
    Gender mainly affected: M = F.
    Etiopathogenesis: VZV.

Diagnostic features

History: After an incubation of 2–3 weeks, primary infection may be subclinical or present with chickenpox. There may be a known epidemic.

Clinical features

Oral: Vesicles, especially in the palate, rupture to produce painful, round or ovoid ulcers, with inflammatory haloes (Figure 10.2).

Extraoral: Centripetal itchy rash (mainly on head, neck and trunk), fever, malaise, irritability, anorexia, cervical lymphadenitis. The rash goes through macular, papular (like "rose petals"), vesicular ("dew drops") and pustular stages, before crusting (Figure 10.3). The rash crops in waves over 2–4 days, and rash fluid is highly contagious but, once lesions scab, they are not. The rash sometimes leaves crater-like scars.

Differential diagnosis: Other viral infections. Smallpox used to be the main differential diagnosis.

Diagnosis is usually clinical. Viral culture, PCR tests, immunostaining or electron microscopy are indicated mainly in immunocompromised patients.

Management

Paracetamol helps analgesia and to reduce fever. Products containing aspirin must not be given to children with chickenpox, as this risks causing the serious and potentially fatal Reye's syndrome (fatty liver and encephalopathy). Antihistamines and calamine lotion may ameliorate itching.

Immune globulin or aciclovir may be indicated in adults, pregnant women, neonates or immunocompromised patients. Valaciclovir or famciclovir may be needed for aciclovir-resistant infections.

Prognosis

Manifestations are generally most severe in adults. Complications are uncommon, but pregnant women or people without immunity against VZV, are at highest risk. Complications may include pneumonia, hepatitis, encephalitis and, rarely, myocarditis, glomerulonephritis and hemorrhage. The most common later complication is zoster.

Infection during pregnancy can damage the fetus and cause zoster later in childhood. Infection in the first 28 weeks of pregnancy, can lead to the fetal varicella syndrome of:
- neurological damage (to brain, eye, spinal cord)
- malformations (toes, fingers, anus and bladder)

Infection late in gestation or immediately postpartum (following birth) may cause neonatal chickenpox, which carries a high risk of pneumonia and other serious complications.

About 75% of deaths from chickenpox are in adults; mortality rates are 2–4 per 100,000.

Zoster (shingles)

Definition: A painful unilateral rash in a dermatome (distribution of a sensory nerve) due to reactivation of VZV latent in the associated sensory ganglion (hence "zoster"; Latin for "belt", since in the thoracic region it causes a strip-like rash).

    Prevalence (approximate): 1–4 cases per year per 1000 healthy adults. Higher in immunocompromised people.
    Age mainly affected: 75% of cases affect people over 50 years. Children may suffer if they are immunocompromised, or if their mother had varicella during pregnancy.
    Gender mainly affected: M = F.
    Etiopathogenesis: VZV reactivation – usually in immunocompromised patients such as those with HIV/AIDS or cancer, or on cancer or immunosuppressive treatments.

Diagnostic features

History: Most zoster is thoracic; 30% affects the trigeminal nerve to cause ipsilateral pain, rash and mouth ulceration in a dermatome (Figure 10.4).

Clinical features

Oral: Unilateral, severe, pain and/or paresthesia occurs before, during and sometimes after (post-herpetic neuralgia, PHN) the rash.

Maxillary zoster – rash over ipsilateral cheek, ulcers and pain in ipsilateral palate and maxillary teeth (Figure 10.5).

Mandibular zoster – rash and pain over lower ipsilateral face and lip, ulcers and pain in tongue, soft tissues and mandibular teeth (Figure 10.6).

Extraoral: Rash is ipsilateral in the dermatome, passing through macular, papular, vesicular and pustular stages before crusting and healing, sometimes with scars. "Zoster sine herpete" describes the rare patient who has all the symptoms except the characteristic rash.

Differential diagnosis HSV

The diagnosis is usually clinical but, if the patient is seen before the rash appears, a misdiagnosis of toothache is possible. Cytology, viral culture, DNA sequentiation, immunostaining or electron microscopy are indicated mainly in immunocompromised patients (Figure 10.7).

Management

Treatment aims to limit severity and duration of pain, shorten duration of the episode, and reduce complications. Systemic aciclovir (high dose) helps resolve zoster and reduce post-herpetic neuralgia (PHN), especially in immunocompromised patients. Early treatment may reduce PHN. Valaciclovir or famciclovir may be needed for aciclovir-resistant VZV. Analgesics treat mouth ulcers and extraoral painful lesions symptomatically. An urgent ophthalmological opinion must be obtained in ophthalmic zoster to obviate corneal damage.

Prognosis

PHN is more likely and severe, in people over 60, when about one in four develop PHN lasting longer than 30 days. Treatment includes antidepressants, anticonvulsants (e.g. gabapentin or pregabalin), lidocaine patches or capsaicin lotion. Opioids may be required.

Herpes zoster oticus (Ramsay-Hunt syndrome type 2) is caused by VZV reactivation in the geniculate ganglion. The syndrome refers to the combination of facial nerve weakness with rash in the ear and external auditory meatus, impaired taste and moisturization of eyes and mouth.

11 Blisters, skin diseases: Pemphigus

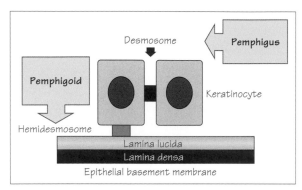

Figure 11.1 Pemphigus compared with pemphigoid.

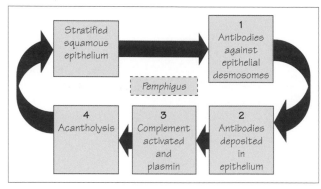

Figure 11.2 Pemphigus pathogenesis.

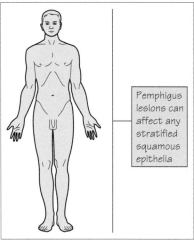

Figure 11.3 Pemphigus affects many epithelia.

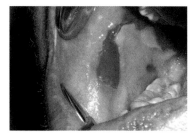

Figure 11.4a Pemphigus showing red lesions.

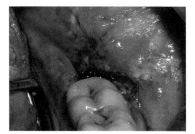

Figure 11.4b Pemphigus lesions.

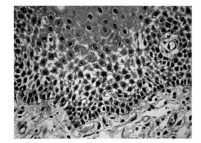

Figure 11.5 Pemphigus acantholysis.

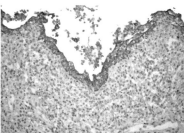

Figure 11.6 Pemphigus basal cells stained with cytokeratin antibody.

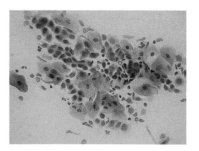

Figure 11.7a Pemphigus Tzanc cells stained by Papanicolaou stain.

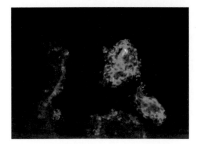

Figure 11.7b Pemphigus IgG staining on acantholytic cells.

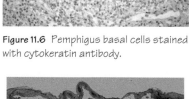

Figure 11.8 Pemphigus intraepithelial blister.

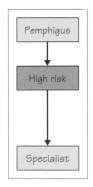

Figure 11.9 Pemphigus treatment.

Several mucocutaneous diseases can present with mouth blisters, erosions, ulcers and/or desquamative gingivitis. Pemphigus is one of the most serious of these diseases since it is potentially lethal, and pemphigoid is of intermediate severity since it can cause blindness and laryngeal scarring. Pemphigus involves damage to desmosomes (causing intra-epithelial blistering); pemphigoid affects hemi-desmosomes (causing sub-epithelial blistering) (Figure 11.1).

Pemphigus

Definition: The term pemphigus originates from the Greek "pemphix" = blister, and is given to a group of autoimmune disorders in which there are autoantibodies directed against components of the desmosomes (epithelial intercellular junctional complex) that enable the keratinocytes to adhere one to another.

Pemphigus vulgaris (PV) is the most common variant; less common variants include pemphigus foliaceus, vegetans, erythematous and paraneoplastic.

Prevalence (approximate): 0.5–3.2 cases per year per 100,000. More frequent among Ashkenazi Jews and, in some rare variants, in South America.

Age mainly affected: Ages 40 to 60.

Gender mainly affected: M = F.

Etiopathogenesis: In PV, autoantibodies directed against the desmosome antigen desmoglein 3 (Dsg 3) attack desmosomes, permitting the cells to separate from each other – a phenomenon termed acantholysis (Figure 11.2).

Dsg1 autoantibodies (the main antigen in pemphigus foliaceus) are also found in over 50% of cases of PV, and the frequency may differ with race since they are found in a significantly greater proportion of patients of Indian origin than white northern Europeans. The proportion of Dsg1 and Dsg3 antibodies appears to be related to site affected and clinical severity; cases of PV which are predominantly oral have only Dsg3 antibodies.

Occasional pemphigus cases are drug-related (e.g. by ACE inhibitors, penicillamine) or occur in myasthenia gravis, lymphoproliferative disorders or inflammatory bowel diseases.

Diagnostic features

History: Soreness and blistering in mouth, other mucosae and skin. PV typically begins in the mouth and can also cause swallowing problems. The blisters usually spread to the skin (Figure 11.3). Hoarseness may also occur if it spreads to the larynx.

Clinical features

Oral: Most pemphigus variants can present with blisters and/or erosions (Figure 11.4a and b) and/or desquamative gingivitis. Oral lesions are the rule in pemphigus vulgaris (PV) but are rare in the superficial and less common pemphigus variants.

Bullae appear on any part of the oral mucosa including the palate, but break so rapidly that they are rarely seen. Usually, the patient presents with large, painful, irregular and persistent red lesions which, by the time they become secondarily infected turn into erosions covered with a yellowish fibrinous slough.

Extraoral: The blisters appear mainly on the skin of the face, back or chest, especially in traumatized areas such as beneath the belt or brassiere, are painful and can erupt, causing raw, crusted wounds. PV usually also affects genitals, and may affect other mucosae.

Differential diagnosis: Pemphigoid, erythema multiforme and other bullous disorders. The Nikolsky sign is more often positive in pemphigus (this is lightly swabbing an unblistered area of skin or mucosa, which if it separates the top layers or causes a blister may indicate pemphigus).

Diagnosis must be confirmed by biopsy and immune studies. There is intraepithelial vesiculation and acantholysis (Figure 11.5), the superficial (upper) portion of the epithelium sloughs off, leaving the bottom layer of cells on the "floor" of the blister which is said to have a "tombstone appearance". Differential binding of anti-desmoglein (anti-Dsg) antibodies suggests that both human skin and monkey esophagus should be used in the diagnosis of PV, since patients with predominantly oral disease may only have Dsg3 antibodies, which are not always detectable using human skin. These antibodies appear as deposits of IgG along with C3 on desmosomes, a pattern reminiscent of chicken wire netting (Figure 11.6), as well as on acantholytic cells (Figures 11.7a and b). There is thus intra-epithelial vesiculation (Figure 11.8).

Anti-Dsg antibodies can be detected in a blood sample by ELISA (Enzyme Linked Immunosorbent Assay), and serum autoantibody titers can help diagnosis and monitoring of disease. A high serum titer of cANCA (cellular AntiNeutrophil Cytoplasmic Antibody) is also seen in PV.

Management

Treatment aims to promote healing of blisters/ulcers, prevent infection, decrease the formation of new lesions and relieve pain. Treatments are most likely to be effective when treatment begins early, before the disease has begun to spread. Specialist care is appropriate (Figure 11.9).

Patients can take steps to reduce the blistering by, for example, avoiding trauma from hard foods and avoiding contact sports or other situations that might cause the skin to blister. Treatment is largely through systemic immunosuppression using corticosteroids, with azathioprine, dapsone, methotrexate, cyclophosphamide, gold or ciclosporin as adjuvants or alternatives. Mycophenolate mofetil offers safer immunosuppression with possibly less nephrotoxicity and hepatotoxicity.

Prognosis

Left untreated, pemphigus is often fatal, usually because of dehydration or infection. Mucosal lesions are recalcitrant, and they may persist even though skin lesions are controlled, and topical corticosteroids or tacrolimus may then help. Anti-B-cell antigen-CD20 monoclonal antibody, rituximab, combined with immune globulin may be an effective alternative therapy for the treatment of refractory PV.

12 Blisters, skin diseases: Pemphigoid

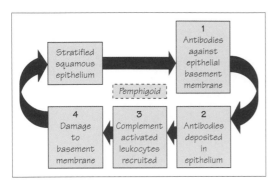

Figure 12.1 Pemphigoid pathogenesis.

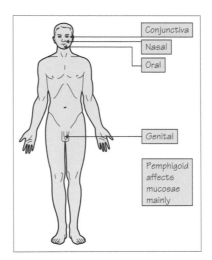

Figure 12.2 Pemphigoid.

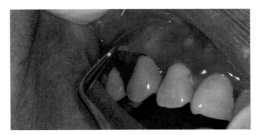

Figure 12.3a Pemphigoid blistering.

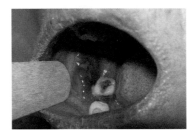

Figure 12.3b Pemphigoid erosions.

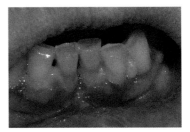

Figure 12.3c Pemphigoid desquamative gingivitis.

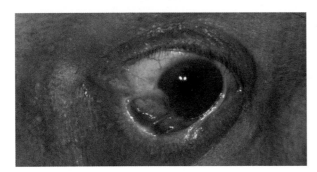

Figure 12.4 Pemphigoid symblepharon.

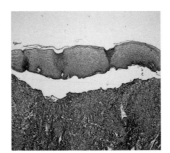

Figure 12.5 Pemphigoid subepithelial blistering.

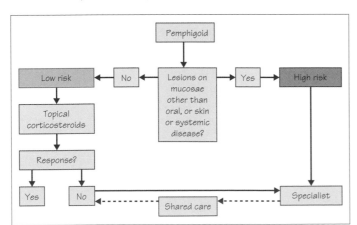

Figure 12.6 Pemphigoid treatment.

24 **Chapter 12** Pemphigoid

Definition: Pemphigoid is the term given to a group of autoimmune disorders which clinically mimic pemphigus but are not lethal. In these conditions there is subepithelial vesiculation, with immune deposits at the epithelial basement membrane zone (EBMZ), rather than acantholysis (Figure 12.1). This spectrum of conditions is termed immune-mediated subepithelial bullous diseases (IMSEBD) and all can present with a similar clinical picture of oral blisters and/or erosions and/or desquamative gingivitis, occasionally with lesions of skin and/or other mucosae (mainly genitals and eyes), and sometimes with scarring.

Prevalence (approximate): Uncommon.

Age mainly affected: Older than 50 years.

Gender mainly affected: F > M.

Etiopathogenesis: A number of pemphigoid variants can affect the mouth, including:

• *Mucous membrane pemphigoid* (MMP) – characterized by oral lesions, sometimes with eye, genital or skin lesions.

• *Oral pemphigoid* (OP) – characterized by oral lesions almost exclusively with autoantibodies to specific molecules in the EBMZ. Many OP patients possess circulating autoantibodies against bullous pemphigoid antigen BP180 (type XVII collagen); in others against alpha 6 integrin, a 120-kDa protein or epiligrin (laminin-5). Patients with antibodies to alpha 6 integrin may have a possible reduced relative risk for developing cancer.

• *Cicatricial pemphigoid* (CP) – may be associated with HLA-DQB1*0301. Different EBMZ components have been implicated, including BP1, BP2, laminin 5 (epiligrin), laminin 6, type VII collagen, beta 4 integrin, and others (uncein, and 45-kDa, 168-kDa and 120-kDa proteins). There may be an association between anti-epiligrin CP and lung carcinoma. A very few cases are drug-induced (e.g. by furosemide or penicillamine)

Diagnostic features

History: Bullae are subepithelial and persist longer than those of pemphigus. Oropharyngeal involvement may present with hoarseness or dysphagia. Progressive scarring may lead to esophageal stenosis. Supraglottic involvement may lead to airway compromise. Nasal involvement may manifest as epistaxis, bleeding after blowing the nose, nasal crusting, and discomfort. Ocular involvement may present with pain or the sensation of grittiness in the eye and conjunctivitis. The perianal area or the genitalia may be blistered or ulcerated (Figure 12.2). Skin lesions are tense vesicles or bullae that may be pruritic and/or hemorrhagic. Scalp involvement may lead to alopecia.

Clinical features

Oral: The oral lesions affect especially the gingivae and soft palate but rarely the vermilion, and may include vesicles or desquamative gingivitis (one of the main manifestations). Tense bullae or vesicles, particularly seen on the soft palate and gingivae, may be blood-filled and remain intact for several days (Figures 12.3a–c). Persistent irregular erosions or ulcers appear after the blisters burst. Oral lesions may scar but this is uncommon. The desquamative gingivitis is typically rather patchy and there is usually persistent soreness (but some cases are asymptomatic).

Extraoral: Eye lesions are the most important. Erosions may be seen on the conjunctivae leading to conjunctival keratinization. Later, entropion develops (eyelids fold inward) with subsequent trichiasis (inturned eyelashes) causing damage to the cornea. With progressive scarring, patients may develop symblepharon (scarring tethering the bulbar and conjunctival epithelia) (Figure 12.4), synechiae (adhesion of the iris to the cornea or lens), and ankyloblepharon (a fixed globe). Lacrimal gland and duct involvement leads to decreased tear production, ocular dryness and further eye damage. The end result of ocular pemphigoid can be eye opacification and blindness.

Nasal involvement may be seen as erosions and crusting in the nasal vestibule. Laryngeal involvement may cause stenosis.

Genital involvement is as painful erosions involving the clitoris, labia, or the glans or shaft of the penis. Perianal involvement manifests as blisters and erosions.

Skin tense blisters or erosions may be seen on either normal-appearing skin or erythematous plaques, most commonly affecting the scalp, head, neck, distal extremities, or trunk.

Differential diagnosis: Differentiate from other causes of mouth ulcers, especially pemphigus vulgaris, lichen planus, IMSEBD (epidermolysis bullosa acquisita, dermatitis herpetiformis and linear IgA disease), localized oral purpura (angina bullosa hemorrhagica), and superficial mucoceles.

Horizontal or tangential pressure to the skin may cause the blister to spread (Nikolsky sign) but this is not a specific sign. Biopsy/histopathology (including immuno-staining) is essential and usually shows subepithelial vesiculation with linear deposits of IgG and sometimes C3 at the basement membrane zone (Figures 12.5).

Serum autoantibodies to epithelial basement membrane may be detected in a few patients.

For evaluation of the upper airway or esophagus, CT scans, barium swallows, or other studies may be helpful and, in patients with anti-epiligrin CP, may be required as part of the search for malignancy.

Management

Treatment aims to suppress extensive blister formation, to promote healing, and to prevent scarring (Figure 12.6). Topical corticosteroids usually help if the lesions are restricted to the oral mucosa but these may need to be potent topical agents such as clobetasol or fluocinolone acetonide cream used for five minutes twice daily or, for the treatment of desquamative gingivitis, in a vacuum formed splint at night. Tetracyclines with or without nicotinamide may help. Dapsone may be useful, especially in the treatment of desquamative gingivitis. Recalcitrant or widespread pemphigoid may respond to tacrolimus, systemic corticosteroids, azathioprine, mycophenolate mofetil, intravenous immunoglobulins or infliximab. An ophthalmological opinion is often indicated.

Prognosis

Without treatment, pemphigoid may persist, with periods of remission and flare-ups, for many years. With treatment, the immune response and inflammation can be suppressed.

13 Pigmented lesions

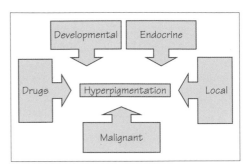

Figure 13.1a *Causes of pigmentation.*

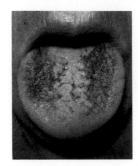

Figure 13.2 Bismuth induced black tongue.

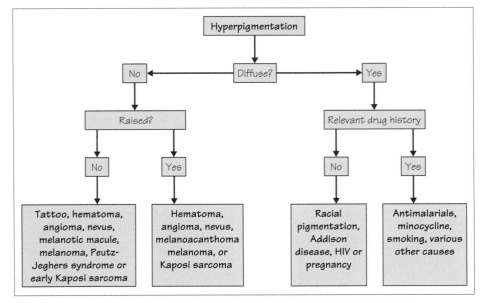

Figure 13.1b *Pigmentation diagnosis.*

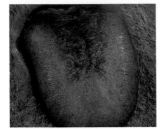

Figure 13.3a Hairy tongue. Note central discoloration.

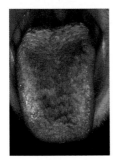

Figure 13.3b *Hairy tongue.*

Table 13.1 *Causes of isolated hyperpigmented lesions.*

Lesion	Main locations	Usual age of presentation	Approximate size	Other features
Amalgam tattoos	Floor of mouth or mandibular gingivae	>5 years	<1 cm	Macular, grayish or black
Graphite tattoos	Palate	>5 years	<0.5 cm	Macular, grayish or black
Kaposi sarcoma	Palate or gingivae	>puberty	Any	Macular, purple or brown, becoming nodular
Melanoma	Palate	Any	Any	Initially macular, brown, gray or black
Melanotic macules	Lips or gingivae	Any	<1 cm	Mostly in caucasians. Macular brown or black
Nevi	Palate	3rd–4th decade	<1 cm	Mostly raised and blue or brown
Purpura	Palate or buccal mucosa	Any	Any	Macular, purple or brown

The oral mucosa is usually not very pigmented despite the fact that it has the same melanocyte density as skin. Pigmentation may be superficial (extrinsic) or intrinsic, isolated lesions or generalized, and ranges from light brown to blue-black, gray, red, or purple – the color depending on the pigment and its depth. Melanin pigment is brown, but can impart a black, brown, blue, or green color to the eye. Vascular lesions tend to be red, purple or blue, but hemorrhage can lead to red, purple, brown or other colors (Tables 13.1 and 13.2).

Intrinsic hyperpigmentation can have a range of causes (Figures 13.1a and b).

Superficial discoloration

Superficial brown discoloration of tongue and teeth, which is easily removed and of little consequence is commonly caused by habits (e.g. cigarette smoking, tobacco or betel chewing); beverages (e.g. coffee, tea and red wine); foods (e.g. beet, liquorice); or by drugs (e.g. iron,

Table 13.2 Causes of oral pigmentation.

Causes	Comments
Drugs and poisons	Iron and chlorhexidine – commonly cause brown staining Antimalarials – yellow (mepacrine) to blue-black (amodiaquine) Minocycline – blue-gray gingival pigmentation caused by staining of the underlying bone Busulphan, other cytotoxic drugs, oral contraceptives, hydroxychloroquine, phenothiazines, anticonvulsants, zidovudine and clofazimine – brown pigmentation Gold – purplish gingival discoloration Heavy-metal poisoning (lead, bismuth and arsenic) now rare, produced black pigmentation
Endocrinopathies	Addison disease
Habits	Betel chewing Tobacco chewing Smoking tobacco is a fairly common cause (smoker's melanosis or intrinsic pigmentary incontinence), with pigment cells appearing in the lamina propria, especially in reverse smoking, practiced in some Asian communities
Melanotic lesions	Melanoma Melanotic macules Nevi
Pregnancy	Sometimes termed chloasma
Racial	Most common cause of hyperpigmentation
Tattoos	Amalgam, graphite, ink, dyes, carbon
Vascular lesions	Kaposi sarcoma Purpura Trauma

chlorhexidine, bismuth) (Figure 13.2). Hairy tongue, often referred to as black hairy tongue, may also appear brown, white, green, or pink.

Hairy tongue (black hairy tongue; lingua villosa nigra)

Definition: Superficial black staining of the dorsum of tongue.

Prevalence (approximate): From 8% in children/young adults to 60% in drug abusers.

Age mainly affected: Older people.

Gender mainly affected: M > F.

Etiopathogenesis: Children rarely have a furred tongue in health but it may be coated with off-white debris in febrile and other illnesses.

Adults, however, not infrequently have a tongue coating in health, particularly if they are edentulous. The filiform papillae are excessively long (normal papillae are < 1 mm in length), and stained by the accumulation of epithelial squames, food debris and chromogenic micro-organisms. The dorsum of tongue is the main oral reservoir of micro-organisms such as *Candida albicans* and viridans streptococci, and those implicated in oral malodor (Chapter 59).

Occasionally, a brown hairy tongue may be caused by drugs that induce xerostomia, or antimicrobials, when it may be related to overgrowth of micro-organisms such as *Candida* spp.

Black hairy tongue is more likely to be seen in those who are:
- edentulous
- on a soft, non-abrasive diet
- poor at oral hygiene
- smokers
- fasting
- febrile
- xerostomic (e.g. Sjögren syndrome or after irradiation).

It is seen particularly in people with poor oral hygiene and who are:
- drug abusers (alcohol, crack cocaine)
- smokers
- betel chewers – when a brownish-red discoloration on the buccal mucosa with an irregular surface that has a tendency to desquamate (and teeth), is seen mainly in women from South and South-East Asia; the epithelium is often hyperplastic, and brownish amorphous material may be seen both on the surface, intracellularly and intercellularly, with epithelial cell ballooning
- eating or drinking highly colored foods (beetroot, black, blue, purple or red berries, confectionery such as liquorice) and drinks (coffee, tea, red wine, exotic alcoholic drinks (with green, blue or purple dyes))
- HIV infected
- have had head and neck radiotherapy

Occasionally other drugs appear responsible (Box 13.1).

Diagnostic features

History: Normally asymptomatic.

Clinical features

Oral: The dorsum of tongue in the central posterior part of the anterior two-thirds (the oral tongue), but never the ventrum, is affected (Figures 13.3a and b). There may also be black or brown superficial teeth staining and, sometimes, oral malodor.

Extraoral: coloured foods, drinks and drugs may also discolor the feces.

Differential diagnosis: Rarely tongue necrosis in giant cell arteritis presents with black discoloration.

Investigations: Rarely indicated.

Management

Discontinue any responsible drugs, mouthwashes, or habits; increase oral hygiene; scrape or brush the tongue in the evenings; use sodium bicarbonate, peroxide or 40% urea in water, chew gum, and/or suck pineapple or a peach stone.

Trichloracetic acid or podophyllum resin or retinoic acid may rarely be needed in recalcitrant cases.

Prognosis

Hairy tongue is not harmful.

Box 13.1 Drugs that may cause black hairy tongue.

- antibiotics (broad spectrum and griseofulvin)
- bismuth-containing preparations
- chlorhexidine
- corticosteroids
- hormone replacement therapy
- iron salts
- MAOI antidepressants
- methyldopa
- perborates
- peroxides
- phenothiazines
- proton pump inhibitors (e.g. omeprazole, lansoprazole)
- tricyclic antidepressants.

Pigmented lesions: Ethnic pigmentation and tattoos

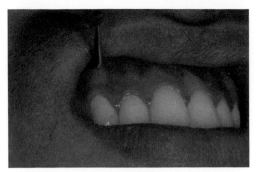

Figure 14.1 Gingival racial pigmentation (very mild).

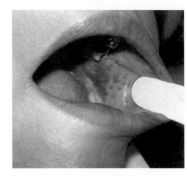

Figure 14.2 Buccal racial melanosis.

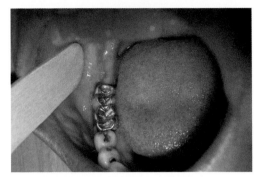

Figure 14.3 Amalgam tattoo.

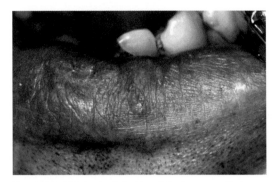

Figure 14.4 Foreign body tattoo following an explosion.

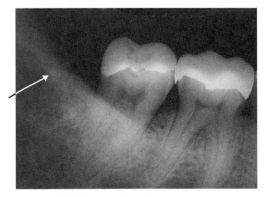

Figure 14.5 Submucosal amalgam may cause amalgam tattoo (patient from Figure 14.3).

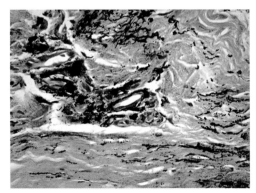

Figure 14.6 Amalgam tattoo × 40.

Ethnic pigmentation

Definition: Physiologic oral pigmentation manifests as multifocal or diffuse melanin pigmentation seen mainly in various ethnic groups, especially people of African or Asian heritage, but can also be noted in patients of Mediterranean descent, sometimes even in quite light-skinned people.

Prevalence (approximate): Occurs in all races. The intensity and distribution of racial pigmentation is variable, not only between races, but also between different individuals of the same race and within different areas of the same mouth.

Age mainly affected: All ages.

Gender mainly affected: M = F.

Etiopathogenesis: The darker a person's skin color the more likely they are to have oral pigmentation. Skin color is a quantitative polygenic trait that varies continuously on a gradient from dark to light. Genes known to contribute to skin color are the MC1R and SLC24A5 genes.

Diagnostic features

History: May be first noticed in adult life and then assumed incorrectly to be acquired rather than congenital.

Clinical features: Brown or blackish patches most obvious in the anterior labial gingivae (Figure 14.1) and palatal mucosa, usually symmetrically distributed. Patches or spots may also be seen on the dorsal tongue, buccal mucosa (Figure 14.2), soft palate or elsewhere. The relative constancy of the color, with no other mucosal change, indicates the benign nature.

Foreign body tattoos

Definition: Tattoos caused by the introduction of colored foreign material.

Prevalence (approximate): Amalgam tattoo affects 1 per 1000 adults.

Age mainly affected: Older adults.

Gender mainly affected: F > M.

Etiopathogenesis: Amalgam, an alloy of mercury, silver, tin, copper and zinc used in dental restorations is the common cause of intraoral "natural" tattoos. Silver is the main culprit. When amalgam is removed with a high-speed dental handpiece, particles can be traumatically implanted in the mucosa, as they can during tooth extraction or root end surgery.

Tattoos may also result from stabbing with a pencil or pen, leaving graphite or ink. Graphite tattoos result from pencil lead traumatically implanted, usually during a childhood accident. Tattoos can also occur with substances like gunpowder, lead shot and bullets or when a substance such as asphalt is introduced into a wound in a road accident or trauma. Coal miners may develop characteristic tattoos.

Some people may also choose to be tattooed for cosmetic, religious, cultural or sentimental reasons, or to symbolize their belonging to, or identification with, particular groups, including a particular ethnic group, criminal gangs or even law-abiding subculture. Men are just slightly more likely to obtain a tattoo than are women.

Many different pigments and dyes are used to make these tattoos, from inorganic materials like ash, to titanium dioxide, iron oxide, carbon, azo dyes, naphthol, phthalocyanine, quinolone, and plastics such as polymethyl methacrylate (PMMA) or ABS (acrylonitrile butadiene styrene).

Diagnostic features

History

Oral tattoos are usually symptomless and rarely enlarge significantly. Older persons with these tattoos may not be able to recall the causal event.

Clinical features

Oral: Amalgam tattoo usually presents as a solitary, soft, painless, non-ulcerated, blue/gray/black macule with no surrounding erythematous reaction, most frequently found on the mandibular gingival or alveolar mucosa (Figure 14.3), but many cases are seen on the lateral tongue, or buccal mucosa. The tattoo is only moderately demarcated from the surrounding mucosa and is usually less than 0.5 cm in greatest diameter, although rare examples have been > 3.0 cm.

In those who exhibit a strong macrophage response to the material, the discolored patch can enlarge over time as the macrophages engulf the foreign material and attempt to move it out of the area.

Graphite tattoos are typically gray-black, often macular, commonly found in the palate, and correspond to the size of the implanted lead or the rub from its introduction. Other accidental tattoos are most common on the lips (Figure 14.4) and facial skin, and are typically black and multiple macules and sometimes nodules.

Intentional tattoos are readily identifiable, often as vulgarities, letters, or symbols in the labial or lingual mucosa, and they are often deeply pigmented with a variety of colors.

Differential diagnosis: Melanotic macule, melanoma, nevus and melanoacanthoma.

Investigations

Lesions with larger particles may be visible on intraoral dental radiographs (Figure 14.5; this shows the same patient as in Figure 14.3).

Biopsy/histopathology is rarely indicated unless to exclude melanoma. Submucosal clusters of small black/brown rounded particles often coat blood vessels and reticulin fibers, staining tissue just as silver histological stain would (Figure 14.6). Occasional larger, angular particles are seen, often surrounded by dense fibrous connective tissue. The stroma around freshly embedded particles shows neovascularity and a pronounced inflammatory cell response. Otherwise, an inflammatory response is rare, and when present, more often in smaller particles, is usually of chronic inflammatory cells. If histiocytes and foreign body multinucleated giant cells are associated with the particles, the lesion is said to be a foreign body reaction. Occasionally amalgam deposits are found in bone, especially after its deliberate placement into the root apical canal during endodontic surgery. These particles may cause black discoloration of the adjacent bone.

Management

Lesions visible on radiographs are usually not biopsied or treated.

Biopsy may be indicated to exclude a melanoma, and those visible on the vermilion of the lips are usually removed also for esthetic reasons.

Prognosis

Tattoos have no malignant potential.

15 Pigmented lesions: Melanotic macule

Benign lesions similar microscopically to racial pigmentation, presenting normal or increased numbers of melanocytes often with subepithelial pigment-laden macrophages (melanophages), and not showing nevi cells thus helping differentiate them from melanocytic nevi, include:
• *Melanotic macules*, which consist of increased melanin, without increased numbers of melanocytes.
• *Ephelides* with sun exposure change in the amount of melanin and consequently color, but melanotic macules do not.
• *Melanoacanthomas* – rare acquired brown to black, usually single, benign areas of pigmentation of the mucosa, which can arise suddenly and enlarge, commonly seen on the buccal mucosa of women of African heritage. Besides increased amount of melanin in the basal layer they also typically show dendritic cells with melanin and eosinophils in the upper epithelium. They may be melanotic macules that appear suddenly as reactive lesions following trauma.

Melanotic macule

Definition: Melanotic macule is an acquired, small, flat, brown to brown-black, asymptomatic, benign lesion, unchanging in character.

Prevalence (approximate): 1 in 1000 adults.

Age mainly affected: Adults.

Gender mainly affected: F > M.

Etiopathogenesis: The oral melanotic macule is a focal increase in melanin deposition. Labial melanotic macule (on the lip vermilion) is regarded as a distinct entity.

Melanotic macules are usually seen in isolation but may also be seen in:
• *Peutz-Jeghers syndrome* – an autosomal dominant trait related to serine/threonine kinase gene, characterized by mucocutaneous melanotic macules, especially circumorally and hamartomatous intestinal polyposis mainly in the small intestine, which rarely undergo malignant change but can produce intussusception (obstruction). The risk of gastrointestinal, pancreatic, breast and reproductive carcinomas is slightly increased.

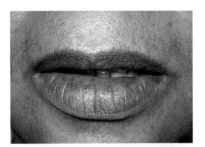

Figure 15.1a Laugier-Hunziker syndrome lip.

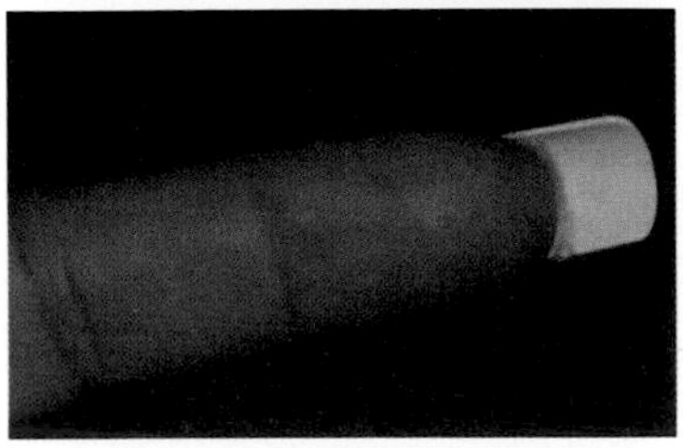

• *Laugier–Hunziker syndrome* – a benign condition of labial, oral, skin and nail hyperpigmentation (Figures 15.1a and b). Genital involvement is not uncommon.
• *HIV infection* – most are related to primary adrenocortical deficiency or to zidovudine therapy.

Diagnostic features

History

Asymptomatic oral melanotic macules unchanging in character.

Clinical features

Most are solitary and seen in white adults and their color ranges from brown to black. Many macules occur on the vermilion border of the lower lip as solitary lesions (labial melanotic macules). Intraorally, the anterior gingivae, buccal mucosa, and palate are the main sites, and more than one lesion may be detected (Figures 15.2 and 15.3). The typical macule is a small well-demarcated, uniformly tan to dark brown, round or oval discoloration < 7 mm diameter.

Differential diagnosis: Tattoos, nevi, melanoma.

Biopsy/histopathology may be indicated if the lesion clinically resembles early melanoma, especially if it develops rapidly. Histopathologically, the stratified squamous epithelium is normal apart from increased pigmentation within the keratinocytes of the basal and parabasal layers, accentuated at the tips of rete ridges. There is negative staining for HMB-45 (homatropine methylbromide) while nevi are positively staining.

There are no nevus cells or elongated rete ridges. There is melanin in the epithelial basal layer and/or upper lamina propria. Deposits may also be seen within subepithelial stroma (melanin incontinence), perhaps within macrophages or melanophages. Brown formalin deposits can be differentiated from iron deposits by their association with erythrocytes rather than with basal layer epithelial cells. There is no underlying inflammatory response.

Management

The intraoral melanotic macule has no malignant transformation potential, but an early melanoma could have a similar clinical appearance, so lesions of recent onset, large size, irregular pigmentation, unknown duration, or enlarging should be excised and examined histopathologically. No treatment is required otherwise, except for cosmetic considerations (excision or removal by laser or hidden by lipstick).

Prognosis

Excellent.

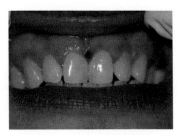

Figure 15.1b Laugier-Hunziker syndrome pigmentation.

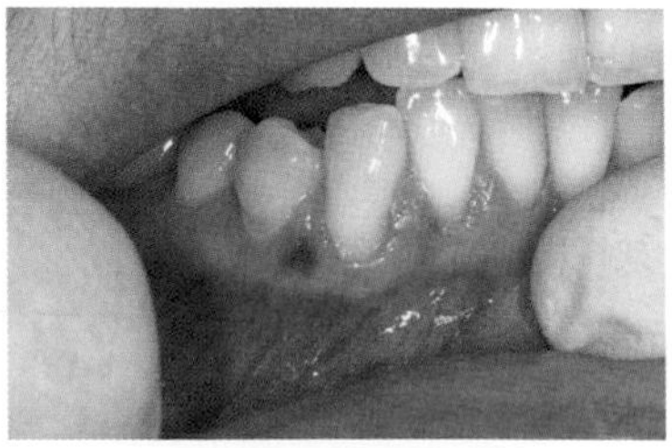

Figure 15.2 Melanotic macules.

Figure 15.3 Melanotic macule.

16 Pigmented lesions: Nevus and others

Definition: Nevus is a broad term that refers to a number of different lesions, often present from birth (from nævus, Latin = birthmark), but can also be acquired. Though the term is also used in reference to hamartomatous or neoplastic entities that are not pigmented (e.g. white sponge nevus), nevus as generally used refers to a melanin pigmented lesion.

Prevalence (approximate): Oral nevi are much less common than cutaneous, occurring in only 1/2000 adults.

Age mainly affected: Nevus frequency increases rapidly in childhood, and peaks in the teens or early twenties and then progressively declines during later life. There are some suggestions that there is a latitude gradient for the age at which the number of nevi peak.

Gender mainly affected: M = F.

Etiopathogenesis: Nevi are formed from increased melanin-containing cells, nevus cells, which are oval/round and are found in unencapsulated nests (theques) either within or beyond the epithelial (mucosal or cutaneous) layer. Melanin production is variable. Nevi include:

• *Intramucosal nevus* (about 60%), consists of a collection of melanocytic cells in the lamina propria without involvement of the epithelium (Figures 16.1a and b).
• *Blue nevus* (25%), deeply situated and are composed of spindled cells at any level in the lamina propria (Figures 16.2a and b).
• *Rare variants*:
  — junctional, consists of clusters of benign nevus cells confined to the basal layer at the epithelial-mesenchymal junction and the lamina propria is otherwise not involved
  — compound nevi (the epithelium and corium) are involved
  — combined nevi

There are many subtypes of nevi, with different clinical and microscopical characteristics; most stain with HMB-45. Nevi tend to mature and pass from junctional to compound and then intramucosal (intradermal) types (by far the most common type), and the cells also mature, acquiring a neuroid aspect. Pigmentation of nevus is variable, even in the same lesion.

Nevi, though usually benign, can be atypical and potentially transform into melanomas, but there is no evidence for this in the mouth

Diagnostic features

History: Nevi are asymptomatic, unchanging in character.

Clinical features: Approximately 85% of oral nevi are pigmented and 15% are amelanotic. Pigmented nevi are seen particularly in the palate (40%), followed by the buccal mucosa (20%) or the vermilion border of the lip. They are usually brown and macular, but compound nevi tend to be papular; they do not change rapidly in size or color and are painless.

Differential diagnosis: Melanotic macules, tattoos, melanoma, melanoacanthoma.

Management

There is no evidence that most pigmented nevi progress to melanoma and though there has been concern that junctional nevi may be a risk factor, evidence does not support this. However, pigmented nevi may resemble melanomas and if early detection of melanomas is to be achieved, all pigmented oral cavity lesions should be viewed with suspicion. Therefore, excision biopsy is recommended; this is particularly important if the lesions are raised or nodular.

Prognosis

Good.

Adenocorticotrophic hormone effects (ACTH)

Oral and skin hyperpigmentation may be seen in ACTH therapy, Addison's disease (adrenocortical hypofunction which results in hypotension, and a feedback pituitary overproduction of ACTH), Nelson syndrome (similar but iatrogenic and results from adrenalectomy in the management of breast cancer) or ectopic ACTH production (e.g. by bronchogenic carcinoma). The brown or black pigmentation is variable in distribution but is usually widespread and seen typically on the soft palate, buccal mucosa (Figure 16.3) and at sites of trauma.

Hyperpigmentation is generalized and brown, and is most obvious in areas normally pigmented, such as the:
• areolae of nipples
• genitalia
• skin flexures
• sites of trauma

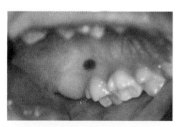

Figure 16.1a Intramucosal nevus.

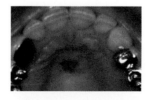

Figure 16.1b Intramucosal nevus.

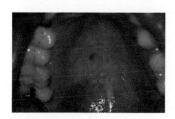

Figure 16.2a Blue nevus.

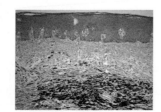

Figure 16.2b Blue nevus.

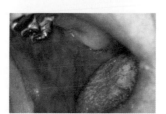

Figure 16.3 Pigmentation in Addison disease.

17 Pigmented lesions: Malignant melanoma

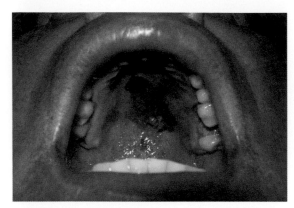

Figure 17.1 Melanoma.

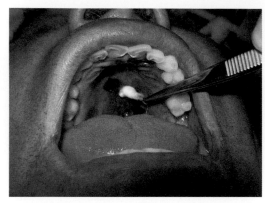

Figure 17.2a Melanoma; testing with cotton pledget.

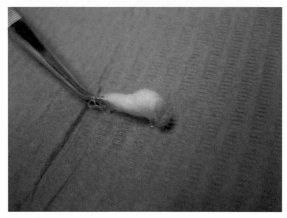

Figure 17.2b Melanoma; cotton is stained.

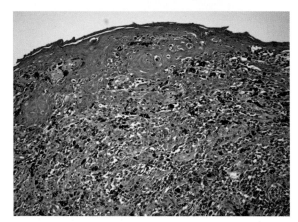

Figure 17.3 Melanoma 10 ×.

Definition: Malignant neoplasm of melanocytes.

Prevalence (approximate): Uncommon – probably 1.2 cases per 10 million population per year. Japan and Uganda are areas of higher prevalence. Oral melanoma accounts for 0.2–8% of melanomas and approximately 1.6% of all head and neck malignancies. The oral mucosa is primarily involved in less than 1% of melanomas.

Age mainly affected: Middle-aged and older.

Gender mainly affected: M > F.

Etiopathogenesis: Sunlight exposure is causal in skin melanomas, which have increased in almost epidemic fashion over the past decades, especially in fair-skinned peoples. The cause of oral melanoma, however, is unknown and no link has been established with chemical or physical trauma, tobacco use, betel chewing or oral hygiene. Most oral melanomas are thought to arise *de novo*. Though oral nevi are potential sources of some melanomas they are usually benign. Even blue nevi, which are more common on the palate – the site of predilection for melanoma – rarely undergo malignant transformation.

Diagnostic features

History: Melanomas are usually symptomless in early stages; later swelling, tooth mobility, or bleeding may appear.

Clinical features

The most common oral locations are the palate and maxillary gingiva. Metastatic melanoma most frequently affects the mandible, tongue, and buccal mucosa.

Oral melanoma often is overlooked or clinically misinterpreted as a benign pigmented process until it is well advanced and it frequently presents with metastases in lymph nodes, liver and lungs. Radial (horizontal spread) and vertical (infiltrative) extension is common at the time of diagnosis.

Pigmented solitary small brown or black macules 1.0 mm to 1.0 cm or larger are found (Figure 17.1). They grow rapidly, initially spreading radially and superficially, later become increasingly pigmented, nodular, deeply invasive and with satellite lesions. Up to 10% are non-pigmented (amelanotic melanoma) and appear as a white, mucosa-colored, or red mass.

Occasionally melanomas are nodular *ab initio* with deep spread, or are multiple or large. Features suggestive of malignancy include a rapid increase in size, change in color, ulceration, pain, bleeding, the occurrence of satellite pigmented spots, or regional lymph node enlargement.

Differential diagnosis: Melanotic macule, nevus, tattoos, melanoacanthoma and Kaposi sarcoma.

Rubbing with a cotton pledget may elicit brown pigmentation (Figures 17.2a and b) but biopsy/histopathology is required (Figure 17.3).

Melanoma histology may show anaplastic spindle-shaped or squamoid cells. The epithelium is abnormal, with large atypical melanocytes and excessive melanin. The melanoma cells have large nuclei, often with prominent nucleoli, and show nuclear pseudoinclusions due to nuclear membrane irregularity. The abundant cytoplasm may be uniformly eosinophilic or optically clear. Occasionally, the cells become spindled, a finding interpreted as a more aggressive feature. However, the histology is quite varied and staining with dopa or antibodies may be required to help the diagnosis. Melanoma stains positively with S100, tyrosinase, Mart-1/melan-A, vimentin, microphthalmic transcription factor, and homatropine methylbromide (HMB-45). Immunohistochemistry, though helpful to differentiate melanoma from other tumors, cannot differentiate from nevus (usually atypical nevus).

Imaging is needed to exclude invasion. Contrast-enhanced CT can be used to determine the extent of the melanoma and whether local, regional, or lymph node metastasis is present. MRI is used to diagnose melanoma in soft tissue. Bone scanning with gadolinium-based agents and chest radiography can be beneficial in assessing metastasis.

Positron emission tomography (PET) has poor results in distinguishing melanoma from nevi. However, combined PET-CT may have diagnostic value.

Management

The optimal treatment is surgery with neck dissection if regional lymph nodes are involved. Prophylactic neck dissection is not advocated as a treatment. Early surgical intervention when local recurrence is detected enhances survival, because dismal outcomes are associated with distant metastasis.

Radiation and chemotherapy are unhelpful. However, although radiation alone is reported to have questionable benefit (particularly in small fractionated doses), it is a valuable adjuvant in achieving relapse-free survival when high-fractionated doses are used. Drug therapies used in the treatment of cutaneous melanoma (dacarbazine in conjunction with interleukin-2 (IL-2)), and immunotherapy, are of questionable benefit in oral melanoma. There are anecdotal reports of benefit from interferon alfa (INF-A). Many centers, however, follow surgery with IL-2 adjunctive therapy to prevent or limit recurrence.

Prognosis

The prognosis is poor and worse than skin melanomas, unless detected very early, but many patients present in advanced stage with involvement of cervical nodes and distant metastases to lung or liver. The five-year survival rate is generally 5–50%. Tumor thickness or volume (Clark and Breslow indices) and lymph node metastasis are less reliable prognostic indicators than they are in skin (where lesions thinner than 0.75 mm rarely metastasize).

18 Red and purple lesions

Red or purple oral lesions are usually caused by increased vascularity or extravasations of blood; pressure with a glass slide (diascopy) typically causes blanching if the lesion is a vascular one (Figure 18.1). Inflammation is the common cause of redness (erythema) but there are other causes (Figure 18.2) (Table 18.1).

For example, chronic gingivitis is the usual cause of gingival redness, usually restricted to the areas inflamed by dental plaque accumulation – gingival margins and interdental papillae. More widespread gingival erythema, particularly if associated with soreness, in children is usually caused by primary herpes stomatitis. In adults the main cause of widespread gingival erythema is desquamative gingivitis (usually due to lichen planus or mucous membrane pemphigoid) (Figure 18.3). Erythema is also occasionally induced by allergic responses (e.g. plasma cell gingivitis). Candidosis can affect large areas and is common, for example, beneath dental appliances, as these alter the local ecology, permitting the yeast to proliferate. Erythema involving large mucosal areas, at any age, may be caused by mucositis, which can cause widespread erythema, erosions and ulcers.

Localized red areas may represent trauma, erythema migrans (Figure 18.4), erythroplasia, carcinoma, candidosis (Figure 18.5), lichen planus, lupus erythematosus or vascular lesions (telangiectasias, varicosities, and hemangiomas) (Figure 18.6). The latter are of red, blue, or purple color due to intravascular blood. Telangiectasia may be a manifestation of hereditary hemorrhagic telangiectasia, primary biliary cirrhosis or scleroderma, or may follow radiotherapy. Hemangiomas are usually seen in isolation but may be part of a syndrome. Some lumps such as pyogenic granulomas may be red (Figure 18.7). Kaposi sarcoma may present as a red, purple, brown or bluish macule or nodule and may be mimicked by epithelioid angiomatosis. The discoloration is due to extravasation of blood, coupled with vascular proliferation. Neither lesion blanches on diascopy.

Blood-filled blisters may be seen in purpura, localized oral purpura (angina bullosa hemorrhagica) and pemphigoid, and occasionally in pemphigus or amyloidosis.

Purpura

Ecchymosis and petechiae, due to bruising and negative pressure (Figure 18.8), are common in the junctional area of the hard and soft palates; they do not blanch with pressure because of blood extravasation. The color can vary from blue, to purple, to red, to brown. The greens and yellows associated with bruises on skin surfaces are not commonly seen intraorally. Petechiae are usually caused by trauma, often from suction, but a bleeding tendency (as in EBV, parvovirus or HIV infections, or idiopathic thrombocytopenic purpura or leukemias) must be excluded.

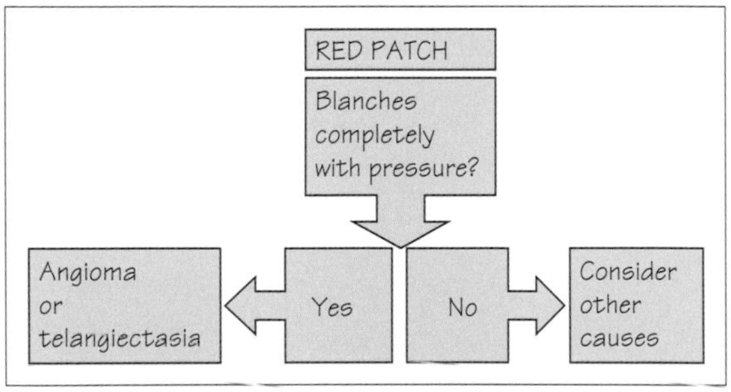

Table 18.1 Causes of red or purple lesions.

Localized	Generalized
Angina bullosa hemorrhagica (blisters)	Candidosis
Angiomas (purple)	Mucosal atrophy (e.g. avitaminosis B)
Avitaminosis B_{12}	Mucositis
Burns	Polycythemia
Candidosis	
Deep mycoses	
Denture-related stomatitis	
Desquamative gingivitis	
Drug allergies	
Erythroplasia	
Geographic tongue	
Granulomatous diseases	
Kaposi sarcoma	
Lichen planus	
Lupus erythematosus	
Purpura	
Telangiectasias	

Figure 18.1 Red lesion diagnosis.

Figure 18.2 Red lesion; causes.

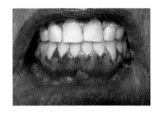

Figure 18.3 Desquamative gingivitis in pemphigus.

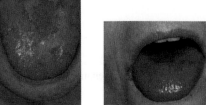

Figure 18.4 Erythema migrans.

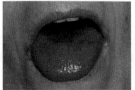

Figure 18.5 Candidosis and angular stomatitis.

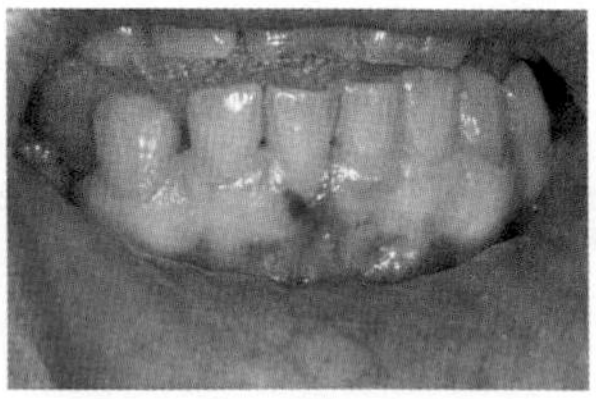

Figure 18.6 Telangiectasia.

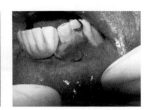

Figure 18.7 Pyogenic granuloma.

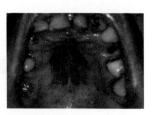

Figure 18.8 Purpura.

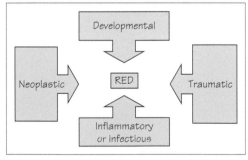

19 Red and purple lesions: Desquamative gingivitis, mucositis

Desquamative gingivitis

Definition: Desquamative gingivitis (previously called gingivosis) is a clinical term for persistently sore, red glazed, or red and ulcerated gingivae.

Prevalence (approximate): Fairly common.

Age mainly affected: Middle-aged or older.

Gender mainly affected: F > M.

Etiopathogenesis: Desquamative gingivitis is not a disease entity but usually a manifestation of atrophic or erosive lichen planus or mucous membrane pemphigoid, and occasionally seen in pemphigus or other dermatoses. It can also be due to sodium lauryl sulfate, allergic reactions, linear IgA or other subepithelial immune blistering diseases, or unknown causes.

Diagnostic features

History

Oral: Persistent gingival soreness, worse on eating, especially spices.

Extraoral: There may be a rash or blisters if the patient has a dermatosis.

Clinical features

Oral: Red and glazed (patchy or uniform) gingivae are seen, especially labially (Figure 19.1). Gingival erythema blurs the distinction between the normally coral pink attached gingivae and the more red vestibular mucosae. The erythema is exaggerated where oral hygiene is poor. Gingival margins and edentulous ridges tend to be spared.

Other oral lesions of dermatoses may be associated (e.g. blisters, erosions or white lesions).

Extraoral: Cutaneous lesions of dermatoses may be associated.

Differential diagnosis: Necrotizing ulcerative gingivitis, plasma cell gingivitis, psoriasis, mechanical chronic trauma.

Investigations: The diagnosis is usually obvious from the history and clinical findings. Nikolsky sign may be positive, but biopsy and immunostaining are often needed to establish the precise cause.

Management

Treatment should be of the underlying condition, and oral hygiene should be maintained. A powered toothbrush may help clean the teeth whilst avoiding gingival trauma, which causes pain.

Topical corticosteroids often help control the inflammation, especially creams used overnight in a polythene splint. If there are extraoral lesions or severe oral ulceration in addition, then systemic therapy, usually with corticosteroids may be required. Other therapies available for recalcitrant lesions include ciclosporin, dapsone, acitretine, sulfapyridine, tetracyclines and tacrolimus.

Prognosis

Good (depends on the underlying disease).

Mucositis

Definition: Mucositis, sometimes called mucosal barrier injury, is the term given to the widespread erythema, ulceration and soreness that commonly complicates a number of therapeutic procedures involving chemotherapy, radiotherapy or chemoradiotherapy, used largely in the treatment of cancer but also in the conditioning prior to bone marrow transplantation (i.e. hematopoietic stem cell transplantation).

Prevalence (approximate): Many patients on chemotherapy develop mucositis – cisplatin, etoposide, fluorouracil and melphalan are particularly implicated. Mucositis invariably follows external beam radiotherapy involving the orofacial tissues, and is also common in upper mantle head and neck radiation, and particularly in total body irradiation. Mucositis is particularly severe after hemopoietic stem cell transplantation, because of the combination of radiation damage and myeloablation.

Age mainly affected: Middle-aged or older.

Gender mainly affected: F = M.

Etiopathogenesis: Damage to the rapidly divided epithelial cells lining the gastrointestinal tract.

Diagnostic features

Mucositis appears 3–15 days after the above treatments, earlier after chemotherapy than after radiotherapy. In chemotherapy, mucositis can occur anywhere along the digestive tract from the mouth to the anus. It typically presents with pain which can be so intense as to interfere with eating and significantly affect the quality of life. The oral mucosa becomes red and thin, may slough and then becomes eroded and ulcerated and sometimes bleeds; the erosions/ulcers often becoming covered by a yellowish white fibrin clot termed a pseudomembrane (Figure 19.2). There is often also disturbed sense of taste. More importantly, the impaired mucosal barrier and immunity in mucositis predispose to life-threatening septic complications.

Management

Prophylaxis of mucositis is the goal; oral cooling with ice chips, keratinocyte growth factor and low-level laser therapy can reduce chemotherapy-induced mucositis. Fractionated radiation dosage increases the risk of radiation-induced mucositis to > 70% of patients in most trials; mucosal shielding may reduce mucositis. One of the goals of targeted cancer therapy (usually monoclonal antibodies or small molecules such as tyrosine kinase inhibitors) is to have treatments with fewer adverse effects than chemotherapy or radiation therapy. Examples of agents used in targeted cancer therapy include rituximab and trastuzumab, cetuximab, erlotinib and gefitinib – oral mucositis from these alone appears uncommon.

The aims of treatment of mucositis are to relieve pain, speed healing and prevent infectious complications. Opioids (i.e. morphine) systemically, and topical benzydamine, barrier protective gels and other agents can reduce pain. Oral hygiene maintenance is important. Monitoring microbial colonization and using antiviral and antifungal prophylaxis, is particularly important in patients with low neutrophil leukocyte counts.

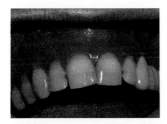
Figure 19.1 Pemphigoid.

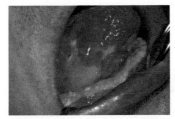
Figure 19.2 Mucositis.

Red and purple lesions: Erythematous candidosis

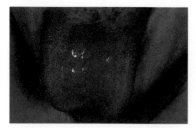

Figure 20.1 Candidal glossitis.

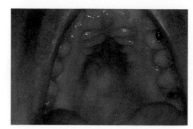

Figure 20.2 Candidal infection in the palate.

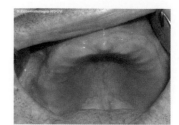

Figure 20.3a Denture related stomatitis.

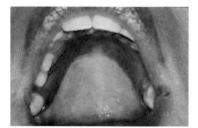

Figure 20.3b Denture related stomatitis.

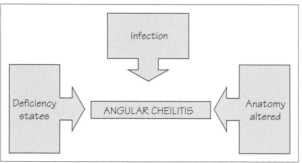

Figure 20.4 Causes of angular cheilitis (angular stomatitis).

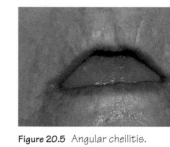

Figure 20.5 Angular cheilitis.

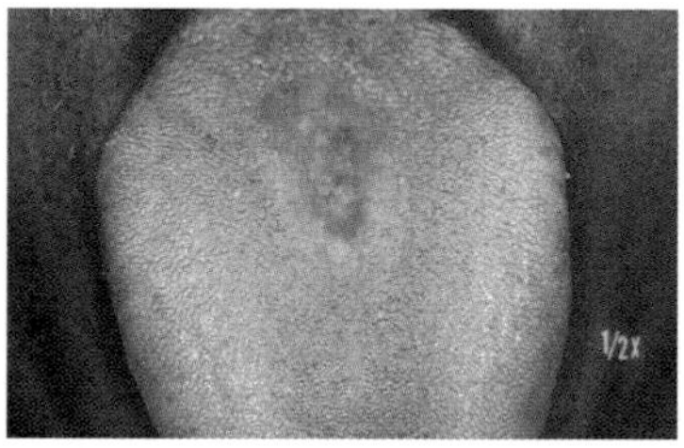

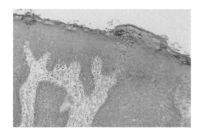

Figure 20.6 Median rhomboid glossitis.

Figure 20.7 Median rhomboid glossitis ×10.

Table 20.1 Types of oral candidosis.

Type	Other terminology	Usual age at onset	Predisposing factors
Acute pseudomembranous	Thrush	Any	Dry mouth, antimicrobials, corticosteroids, immune defect
Acute atrophic	Antibiotic sore mouth	Any	Antibiotics or corticosteroids
Chronic atrophic	Denture-related stomatitis	Adults	Denture wearing
Chronic hyperplastic	Candidal leukoplakia	Middle-aged or older	Tobacco, denture wearing, immune defect
Chronic mucocutaneous	—	First decade	Immune defect
Erythematous	—	Any	Immune defect
Median rhomboid glossitis	—	Third or later decades	Tobacco smoking, denture wearing, immune defect

Candidosis can cause oral erythema and soreness, with or without white lesions of pseudomembranous candidosis (Table 20.1).

Acute candidosis

Definition: Acute infection, typically with *Candida albicans*.
  Prevalence (approximate): Unknown.
  Age mainly affected: Adults.
  Sex mainly affected: M = F.
  Etiopathogenesis: Acute erythematous or atrophic candidosis may complicate corticosteroid or broad-spectrum antimicrobial therapy, HIV infection or immunocompromised states, then often with lesions in the respiratory tract and esophagus. *Candida albicans* is the main pathogen. *Candida* spp. infections have increased greatly in immunocompromised people such as those with HIV/AIDS, when *Candida albicans* may be accompanied by other species (especially *C. krusei*). The most dominant other *Candida* species are *tropicalis*, *glabrata*, *parapsilosis*, and new species such as *dubliniensis*, *africanus* and *inconspicua*. Antifungal resistance is also a clinical challenge.

Diagnostic features

Erythematous candidosis may arise as a consequence of persistent pseudomembranous candidosis when the pseudomembranes are shed, or may develop *de novo*. Lesions on the tongue dorsum often present as depapillated areas (Figure 20.1). Central palatal red areas may resemble a "thumb-print" (Figure 20.2). Angular stomatitis and/or pseudomembranous candidosis can be an associated component.

Diagnosis is clinical, supplemented by smear or culture.

Management

Acute candidosis is best treated with antifungal drugs (nystatin, amphotericin, miconazole or fluconazole). Highly Active Antiretroviral Therapy (HAART) reduces the frequency of candidosis in HIV infection.

Chronic candidosis
Denture-related stomatitis (denture sore mouth; chronic atrophic candidosis)

Definition: Diffuse erythema limited to the dental appliance-bearing mucosa.

Prevalence (approximate): About 7% of the population over 30 years and 15% over 60 years.

Age mainly affected: Middle-aged and older.

Sex mainly affected: F > M.

Etiopathogenesis: Found virtually exclusively only under an upper dental appliance (denture or orthodontic plate). It affects only the mucosa contacting the appliance fitting surface, which highlights that it is not caused by an allergic reaction that would affect any mucosae in contact with the appliance.

Trauma is an unlikely cause, since this is less likely beneath an upper than a lower appliance. It appears to be related to ecological changes, from plaque accumulation (bacteria and/or yeasts) between the appliance and palate.

Various micro-organisms (*Candida albicans* mainly, but occasionally *Streptococcus milleri* and *Klebsiella* spp.) have been implicated.

Dry mouth, diabetes, immunosuppressive therapy or a high-carbohydrate diet and HIV disease occasionally predispose.

Diagnostic features
History
Oral. Usually asymptomatic.

Clinical features
Oral: Diffuse erythema limited to denture-bearing area (Figures 20.3a and b). Classified (Newton classification) into types:

(1) a localized simple inflammation or a pinpoint hyperemia

(2) an erythematous or generalized simple type presenting as more diffuse erythema involving a part of, or the entire, denture-covered mucosa

(3) a granular type (inflammatory papillary hyperplasia) commonly involving the central part of the hard palate and the alveolar ridge

Denture-related stomatitis may be accompanied by angular stomatitis.

Differential diagnosis: Trauma, mucositis.

The diagnosis is clinical.

Management

Dental appliances should be cleaned and disinfected at night, and stored in an antiseptic (1% hypochlorite or 0.2% aqueous chlorhexidine). The mucosal infection is eradicated by brushing the palate and using antifungals and an oral antiseptic which is antifungal, such as chlorhexidine.

Prognosis
Good.

Angular stomatitis (angular cheilitis; perleche)

Definition: Angular stomatitis is inflammation of the skin and contiguous labial mucous membrane at the commissures.

Prevalence (approximate): Up to 2% of adults.

Age mainly affected: Adults.

Sex mainly affected: M = F.

Etiopathogenesis: Most cases in adults are due to mechanical and/or infective causes and denture-related stomatitis is associated. *Candida* or *staphylococci* are isolated from most patients. In children nutritional defects such as riboflavin, folate, iron and malabsorption, or immune defects such as in Down syndrome, diabetes and HIV infection are more prominent causes (Figure 20.4).

Diagnosis

Clinical features are bilateral commissural erythema or fissuring (Figure 20.5). Diagnosis is clinical.

Management

Denture-related stomatitis must be treated, and miconazole or fusidic acid cream applied locally.

Median rhomboid glossitis (central papillary atrophy of the tongue)

Definition: A red, depapillated, rhomboidal area in the midline dorsum of tongue.

Prevalence (approximate): 1 in 300–2000 adults.

Age: Middle age and older.

Gender: M > F (3:1).

Etiopathogenesis: Possibly, a defective posterior dorsal point of fusion of lingual tubercles, represents a focal area of susceptibility to candidosis. Smoking, denture-wearing and, occasionally, immune defects (including HIV and diabetes) predispose.

Diagnostic features
History: Often asymptomatic.

Clinical features: A rhomboidal or oval nodular or macular, usually red area (Figure 20.6) in the posterior midline of the anterior dorsum of the tongue. Multiple oral lesions may occasionally be present, especially a "kissing" lesion in the palatal vault.

Differential diagnosis: Erythroplakia, neoplasm, lingual thyroid, gumma, mycobacterial or deep fungal infection, pyogenic granuloma, and granular cell tumor.

Investigations: Diagnosis is usually clinical, although biopsy may be indicated, since some lesions may clinically simulate a neoplasm. The histology often shows irregular pseudoepitheliomatous hyperplasia (Figure 20.7) that may mimic carcinoma.

Management
Smoking cessation and antifungals are indicated.

Nodular cases are often removed for histopathological study.

Prognosis
Good.

Red and purple lesions: Angiomas

Vascular anomalies of the head and neck, sometimes termed angiomas, are divided into two main categories: Vascular malformations (capillary, venous, lymphatic, and arteriovenous malformations (AVM)) and vascular tumors (hemangioma, kaposiform hemangioendothelioma, and tufted angioma).

(See http://emedicine.medscape.com/article/846692-overview.)

Hemangioma

Definition: A reddish, bluish or purplish soft vascular lesion which blanches on pressure.

Prevalence (approximate): 5 in 1000 adults (extraoral angiomas are seen in 2% of newborns).

Age mainly affected: From childhood.

Gender mainly affected: M > F (2:1).

Etiopathogenesis: Hemangiomas in children are usually benign lesions of developmental origin – hamartomas. In adults they differ; they are usually vascular anomalies.

Diagnostic features

History

Oral: Many hemangiomas appear in infancy, most by the age of two years, grow slowly and, by age ten, the majority have involuted (resolved). In adults, hemangiomas rarely involute spontaneously; rather they typically slowly enlarge.

Clinical features

Oral: Most common on the tongue, buccal mucosa or lip, as painless reddish, bluish or purplish soft lesions (Figure 21.1). Hemangiomas usually blanch on pressure, are fluctuant to palpation, are level with the mucosa or have a lobulated or raised surface. Hemangiomas are at risk from trauma and prone to excessive bleeding if damaged (e.g. during tooth extraction). Occasionally, oral hemangiomas develop phlebolithiasis.

Extraoral: Hemangiomas are typically seen in isolation but a few may be multiple and/or part of a wider syndrome such as Sturge-Weber syndrome (angioma that extends deeply and rarely involves the ipsilateral meninges, producing a facial angioma and epilepsy, sometimes with learning impairment); blue rubber bleb nevus syndrome (BRBNS) (Figure 21.2) is characterized by multiple cutaneous venous malformations in association with visceral lesions, most commonly affecting the GI tract; Maffucci syndrome consists of multiple angiomas with

enchondromas; Dandy–Walker syndrome is a congenital brain malformation involving the cerebellum, or other posterior cranial fossa malformations and facial hemangioma.

Differential diagnosis: Kaposi sarcoma and epithelioid angiomatosis should be excluded.

Investigations: The characteristic feature is that they blanch on pressure, or contain blood on aspiration with a needle and syringe. For large angiomas, angiography may be needed. Oral lesions suspected of being hemangiomatous should not be routinely biopsied; aspiration is far safer. After intravenous administration of contrast medium, enhancement is observed in hemangiomas in areas corresponding to those with high signal on T2-weighted magnetic resonance imaging (MRI).

Management

Most angiomas are small, of no consequence and need no treatment, but if they do for esthetic or functional reasons, they respond well to cryosurgery, laser ablation or intralesional injections of corticosteroids, sclerosing agents or interferon alfa. Very large hemangiomas may need to be treated with ligation or embolization, mainly for cosmetics or if bleeding is troublesome.

Prognosis

Some 50% of hemangiomas present in childhood regress spontaneously, but cavernous types tend to do this less, as do those associated with Sturge-Weber syndrome.

Venous lake (venous varix; senile hemangioma of lip)

This is a bluish-purple soft venous dilatation, 2–10 mm in diameter, usually seen on the lower lip of an older person. It can be excised, but careful cryotherapy, electrocautery, infrared coagulation or treatment with an argon laser can also give good results.

Lymphangioma

Lymphangioma is uncommon in the mouth. At least some are hamartomas and many are of similar structure to hemangiomas and can clinically resemble them, with a "frog-spawn" appearance (Figure 21.2), but they contain lymph rather than blood.

Lymphangiomas are usually solitary and affect the tongue predominantly. They are occasionally associated with cystic hygroma. One study has found blue, domed lymphangiomas on the alveolar ridges of about 4% of newborn black children; 90% are diagnosed before two years of age. These lesions, which were usually bilateral, often regressed spontaneously. There is no sex predilection.

Contrast-enhanced T1-weighted MRI can be used to differentiate between lymphangiomas and deep hemangiomas. Small lymphangiomas need no treatment. Larger lesions may require excision, although cryotherapy, laser therapy and sclerotherapy can be useful and more recently, radiofrequency ablation has been described.

Approximately 70–80% of patients with lymphatic malformations experience infections, often associated with significant increases in the size of lesions. Rapid enlargement of the lesion either as a result of intralesional infection or hemorrhage may lead to airway obstruction; as a result of these concerns, approximately 50% of children with such lesions require tracheostomy.

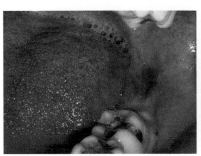

Figure 21.1 Angioma.

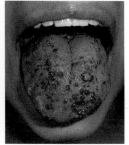

Figure 21.2 Multiple angiomas.

Red and purple lesions: Proliferative vascular lesions, Kaposi sarcoma

Proliferative vascular lesions

Proliferative vascular lesions are common in the head and neck and include:
• Lobular capillary hemangioma (pyogenic granuloma), seen mainly on the gingivae or tongue or lip. Excision suffices.
• Intravascular papillary endothelial hyperplasia (Masson hemangioma or pseudoangiosarcoma), a benign, non-neoplastic, vascular lesion characterized histologically by papillary fronds lined by proliferating endothelium and probably representing an organizing thrombus which may simulate angiosarcoma histologically, is seen especially on the lip. Excision suffices.
• Less common but more aggressive lesions which may be seen include Kaposi sarcoma.
• Rarely seen are epithelioid hemangioma, epithelioid hemangioendothelioma, spindle-cell (kaposiform) hemangioendothelioma, acquired progressive lymphangioma, or angiosarcoma.

Kaposi sarcoma

Definition: Kaposi sarcoma (KS) is not a true sarcoma but a lymphatic endothelial proliferative condition widely regarded as a neoplasm.
   Prevalence (approximate): Uncommon.
   Age mainly affected: Second to fourth decades.
   Gender mainly affected: M > F.
   Etiopathogenesis: KS is induced by human herpesvirus 8 (HHV-8 now termed KSHV – Kaposi sarcoma associated herpesvirus) and is almost exclusively seen in immunocompromised patients. KS was originally described in elderly Jews and those of Mediterranean or Middle Eastern origin (*Classic KS*), in the absence of an identified immune defect but where KSHV infection rates are high. *Endemic KS* was described later in young people, from sub-Saharan Africa (where > 50% are infected with KSHV), as a more aggressive disease. *Transplant related KS* had been described in people on T-lymphocyte inhibitors when a KSHV-infected organ was transplanted, or the recipient had pre-existing KSHV infection. However, a large increase in KS was described during the 1980s, when epidemic KS appeared as an aggressive disease first reported in male homosexuals and eventually recognized to be part of Acquired Immune Deficiency Syndrome (AIDS). KS is over 300 times more common in AIDS patients than in renal transplant recipients. KS is seen when HIV is transmitted sexually; up to 20% of male homosexual AIDS patients have developed oral KS but, in contrast, KS is rare in children with HIV/AIDS.

Diagnostic features

History
Oral: Oral KS is the first presentation of HIV in up to 60% of affected patients. The mouth is the initial site in 15% of AIDS-related KS.

Lesions are often asymptomatic but more than 25% are painful, about 8% bleed, and oral candidosis is often associated.
   Extraoral: KS primarily affects the skin and mucosa in the head and neck, especially the nose.

Clinical features
Oral: KS typically produces a red, bluish, purple, sometimes brown or black, macule (Figure 22.1) which then enlarges to a nodule and may ulcerate. Multiple lesions are common. Up to 95% of lesions are seen in the palate, 23% in the gingiva and others on the tongue or buccal mucosa.
   Extraoral: KS is usually part of widespread disease affecting skin, gastrointestinal, and respiratory tracts.
   Differential diagnosis: From other pigmented lesions, especially hemangiomas, purpura, and epithelioid angiomatosis (bacterial infection with *Rochalimaea henseleae* that responds to antibiotics).

Investigations
KS may be suspected from the lesion appearance and the patient's risk factors, but biopsy is confirmatory, showing spindle cells (Figure 22.2) and KSHV latency-associated nuclear antigen (LANA) in tumor cells, which confirms the diagnosis (Figure 22.3). In the initial stages, KS histologically resembles granulation tissue with dilated vascular spaces, proliferation of endothelial cells and fibroblasts. As KS lesions mature, they become more fibroblastic and spindle cell-like. One of the characteristic features is the vascularity and slit-like vascular spaces which contain erythrocytes which may extravasate, with hemosiderin deposition.
   HIV serology may be indicated after appropriate counseling.

Management
Oral KS often responds to radiotherapy, cryotherapy or to etoposide or vinca alkaloids systemically or intralesionally or, in HIV infected patients, to Anti-Retroviral Therapy (ART). More widespread disease, or disease affecting internal organs, is generally treated with systemic therapy with alfa interferon, liposomal anthracyclines or paclitaxel. Clinical trials are testing antivirals that target KSHV.
   Surgery is rarely recommended, as KS can reappear in wound edges.

Prognosis
With the increased survival among HIV/AIDS patients receiving ART, the incidence and severity of KS also decreased, but KS-associated immune reconstitution following commencement of ART has been reported (IRIS, Chapter 60) and recurrences are not uncommon.

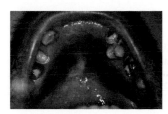

Figure 22.1 Kaposi sarcoma.

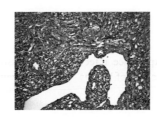

Figure 22.2 Kaposi sarcoma.

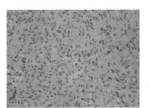

Figure 22.3 Kaposi sarcoma immunostained for KSHV.

Red and purple lesions: Erythroplakia

Table 23.1 Histological terms to describe oral epithelial changes associated with risk of malignancy.

Epithelial dysplasia	Squamous intraepithelial neoplasia (SIN)	Squamous intraepithelial lesions (SIL)
Epithelial hyperplasia		Simple hyperplasia
Mild dysplasia (grade I)	1	Basal/parabasal hyperplasia
Moderate dysplasia (grade II)	2	Atypical hyperplasia
Severe dysplasia (grade III)	3	
Carcinoma in situ		Carcinoma in situ

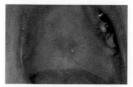

Figure 23.1 Erythroplakia.

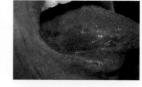

Figure 23.2 Erythroplakia.

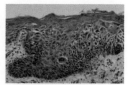

Figure 23.3 Erythroplakia showing dysplasia.

Table 23.2 Cytological and architectural features of epithelial dysplasia.

Cytological	Architectural
Abnormal variation in nuclear size and shape (anisonucleosis and pleomorphism)	Loss of polarity
Abnormal variation in cell size and shape (anisocytosis and pleomorphism)	Disordered maturation from basal to squamous cells
Increased nuclear/cytoplasmic ratio	Includes top-to-bottom change of carcinoma in situ
Enlarged nuclei and cells	Increased cellular density
Hyperchromatic nuclei	Basal cell hyperplasia
Increased mitotic figures	Dyskeratosis (premature keratinization and keratin pearls deep in epithelium)
Abnormal mitotic figures (abnormal in shape or location)	Bulbous drop-shaped rete pegs
Increased number and size of nucleoli	Secondary extensions (nodules) on rete tips

Adapted from Speight PM (2007). Update on oral epithelial dysplasia and progression to cancer. Head and Neck Pathology, 1, 61–66.

Atrophic lesions are characterized by epithelial atrophy and/or absence of keratin production, which means that the underlying vascular lamina propria appears red clinically.

Erythroplakia is the most potentially malignant of all oral mucosal lesions, but is a far less common lesion than leukoplakia.

Erythroplakia (erythroplasia)

Definition: Erythroplakia is defined as "any lesion of the oral mucosa that presents as a bright red velvety plaque which cannot be characterized clinically or pathologically as any other recognizable condition". Erythroplakia is a potentially malignant disorder; almost all lesions contain dysplastic cells and most contain severe dysplasia (40%), or are carcinoma *in situ*, or carcinoma (51%). Carcinomas appear many times more frequently in erythroplakia than in leukoplakia.

Prevalence (approximate): Rare.

Age mainly affected: Older people > 60 years.

Sex mainly affected: M > F.

Etiopathogenesis: Tobacco, alcohol and betel are often implicated. A more than additive interaction has been found between tobacco chewing and low vegetable intake, whereas a more than multiplicative interaction has been found between alcohol drinking and low vegetable or fruit intake.

Diagnostic features

History

Oral: Often symptomless.

Clinical features

Oral: Erythroplakia is typically a single velvety red plaque, usually level with or depressed below surrounding mucosa, sometimes associated with white patches. It is seldom multicentric and rarely covers extensive areas of the mouth. Erythroplakia is usually seen on the soft palate (Figure 23.1) or ventrum of the tongue/floor of mouth (Figure 23.2). Erythroplakia is soft on palpation and does not become indurated until invasive carcinoma develops.

Differential diagnosis: Inflammatory and atrophic lesions (e.g. in deficiency anemias, geographic tongue, lichen), lesions of physical trauma, chemical burns and mucositis.

Investigations

Biopsy/histopathology is indicated. Erythroplakia often presents as "carcinoma *in situ*", a term used by some to describe lesions where epithelial dysplasia involves the whole thickness of the epithelium (Figure 23.3). Although terms such as squamous intraepithelial neoplasia (SIN) or squamous intraepithelial lesions (SIL) are sometimes used, the agreed collective histological term *oral epithelial dysplasia*, is used to describe the features of disordered epithelial maturation and proliferation which are often associated with an increased risk of progression to malignancy (Table 23.1). *Mild dysplasia* (grade I) demonstrates proliferation or hyperplasia of cells of the basal and parabasal layers which does not extend beyond the lower third of the epithelium and is not necessarily indicative of malignant potential; it can also be seen in non-neoplastic reactive lesions such as the regenerating epithelium at the edge of an ulcer, or overlying inflammatory lesions such as candidosis. *Moderate dysplasia* (grade II) demonstrates a proliferation of atypical cells extending into the middle one-third of the epithelium. *Severe dysplasia* (grade III) shows abnormal proliferation from the basal layer into the upper third of the epithelium. *Carcinoma in situ*, is the most severe form of epithelial dysplasia, characterized by full thickness cytological and architectural changes.

Pathologists make an essentially subjective judgment of the degree of dysplasia based on varying combinations of a diverse range of histological features which include:

(1) Irregular hyperplasia (increased cell numbers) particularly of cells with a basal cell morphology (basal cell hyperplasia).

(2) Rete ridges showing a drop-shaped configuration is also a feature of severe dysplasia.

(3) Loss of polarity of cells and loss of normal stratification of the epithelial layer.

(4) Nuclear changes such as an increased nuclear-cytoplasmic ratio, more intense nuclear staining (hyperchromatism) and variations in shape and size (pleomorphism).

(5) Mitoses in upper levels of the epithelium, excess numbers or abnormal mitoses such as triradiate forms.

(6) Individual cell keratinization often in the deep layers (dyskeratosis or premature keratinization).

(7) Loss of intercellular cohesion so that cells tend to separate and in extreme cases are acantholytic (malignant acantholysis) (Table 23.2).

Management

Although dysplastic lesions can regress, the risk of progression to overt malignancy increases with the degree of dysplasia. Thus, erythroplakia should be excised and the patient should be advised to stop tobacco/alcohol/betel habits, and encouraged to have a diet rich in fruit and vegetables.

Prognosis

Long-term monitoring is needed.

Red and purple lesions: Erythema migrans (lingual erythema migrans; benign migratory glossitis; geographical tongue; continental tongue)

24

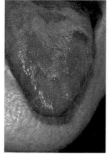

Figure 24.1 *Geographical tongue.*

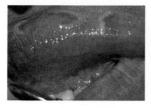

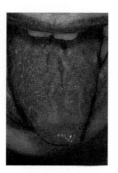

Figure 24.2 *Geographical tongue – erythema migrans.*

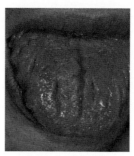

Figure 24.3 *Geographical and fissured tongue.*

Figure 24.4 *Fissured and geographical tongue.*

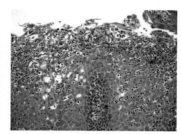

Figure 24.5 *Geographical tongue.*

Oral erythema migrans is a condition absolutely distinct from cutaneous erythema chronicum migrans, which refers to the rash often seen in the early stage of Lyme disease.

Definition: A benign inflammatory condition of the tongue with map-like areas of erythema which are not constant in size, shape or location.

Prevalence (approximate): 1–3% of the population.

Age mainly affected: More prominent in adults than in children.

Gender mainly affected: F > M.

Etiopathogenesis: It appears to be a genetic condition. A positive family history may be obtainable but HLA findings have been equivocal, with reported associations with B15, DR7, DRW6 and CW6. Fissured tongue is often associated.

Diagnostic features

History

Oral: May be asymptomatic or cause a sore tongue. The condition may cause some soreness, especially with acidic foods (e.g. tomatoes). A few relate the oral lesions to other foods, for example spices or cheese, eggplant, walnuts, or citrus. Chemicals, such as some toothpastes, mouthwashes and teeth whiteners, can also cause discomfort.

Patients of any age may be affected but why the condition sometimes gives rise to symptoms after it has been present asymptomatically for decades is unclear.

Extraoral: Some patients with lingual erythema migrans have atopic allergies such as hay fever. Rarely there is an association with:
- pustular psoriasis
- Reiter syndrome
- atopic dermatitis
- pityriasis rubra pilaris.

Clinical features

Oral: Migrating areas of depapillation are seen on the dorsum of the tongue.

Map-like red areas, which are not constant in size, shape or location, with increased thickness of intervening filiform papillae, result in red patches of desquamation surrounded by a yellow border. Alternatively, there are rounded, sometimes scalloped, reddish areas with a whitish margin (Figures 24.1 and 24.2). These patterns change in shape, increase

in size, and spread or move from day to day and even within a few hours. Seen mainly on the dorsum of the tongue, other sites, such as the labial or palatal mucosa can be affected – but only rarely.

Erythema migrans is often found in patients who have a fissured tongue (Figures 24.3 and 24.4).

Differential diagnosis: Lichen planus, lupus erythematosus, candidosis, psoriasis, reactive arthritis (Reiter syndrome) or deficiency glossitis.

No investigations are usually needed unless there is the possibility of deficiency glossitis, diabetes, Reiter syndrome, psoriasis or other disorders.

Biopsy/histopathology is not indicated but shows epithelial thinning at the centre of the lesion, with an inflammatory infiltrate mainly of polymorphonuclear leukocytes (Figure 24.5). There is usually loss of the filiform papillae and a variable inflammatory infiltrate in the corium which is often minimal. Neutrophils are seen, usually in the upper stratum spinosum, scattered or aggregated into micro-abscesses (spongiform pustules) which are characteristic but not pathognomonic as may be seen in psoriasis (where they form micro-abscesses of Munro), Reiter syndrome, plasma cell gingivitis and candidosis. Indeed, whenever spongiform pustules are seen in the upper epithelium the pathologist should look for candidal hyphae with the PAS stain or with a silver stain such as Grocott, because candidosis is one of the most common causes of this.

It may be impossible to distinguish geographical tongue from psoriasis in the absence of a clinical history or extraoral manifestations, and many believe that geographical tongue is a "forme fruste" (an atypical or attenuated manifestation) of psoriasis.

Management

Medical: No effective treatment is available except reassurance, but benzydamine hydrochloride 0.15% spray or mouthwash or topical steroids may provide relief. Zinc or vitamin B are advocated by some and may occasionally help.

Prognosis

There are no complications. Spontaneous resolution of the lesion in one area is not uncommon, but usually another lesion appears in another location.

Swellings: Hereditary conditions, drug-induced swellings

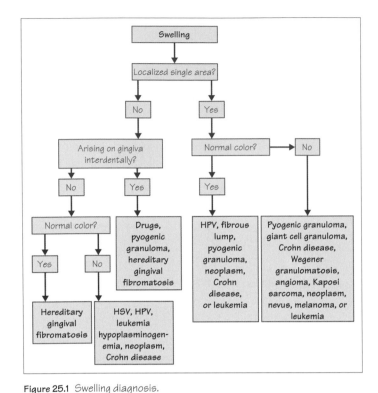

Figure 25.1 Swelling diagnosis.

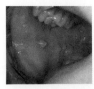

Figure 25.2 Fibrous lump.

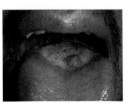

Figure 25.3 Venous malformation (cavernous hemangioma).

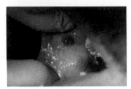

Figure 25.4 Pyogenic granuloma.

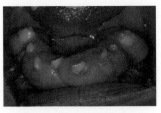

Figure 25.5 Idiopathic gingival fibromatosis.

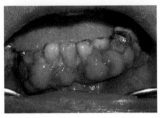

Figure 25.6 Gingival overgrowth from hydantoins.

Table 25.1 Causes of orofacial soft tissue swelling.

Hereditary conditions	Hereditary gingival fibromatosis C1 esterase inhibitor deficiency (hereditary angioedema)	
Acquired conditions	Fluid accumulations	Allergic angioedema Hematoma Surgical emphysema Traumatic edema
	Inflammation	Insect bites/stings Cutaneous or oral infections
	Granulomatous disorders	Crohn disease (and orofacial granulomatosis) Leprosy Melkersson-Rosenthal syndrome Sarcoidosis Tuberculosis Wegener granulomatosis
	Drug-induced and other reactive lesions	Denture-induced hyperplasia Drug-induced swelling Fibrous lumps Giant cell lesions Pyogenic granulomas
	Cysts, hamartomas and neoplasms	Angiomas Lymphangiomas Various cysts Various neoplasms
	Foreign bodies	Any
	Endocrine, metabolic and deposits	Acromegaly Amyloidosis Myxedema Nephrotic syndrome Systemic corticosteroid therapy

Table 25.2 Swellings of different colors.

Color	Examples
Normal pink	Angioedema Drug-induced gingival swelling Epulis fissuratum Familial gingival fibromatosis Fibroma Fibrous lumps (Figure 25.2) Granulomatous disorders Neoplasms Papillomas Warts
Blue	Angioma Eruption cyst Giant cell granuloma Kaposi sarcoma Mucocele Ranula
Black	Melanoma, nevi
Brown	Nevi
Purple	Angioma (Figure 25.3) Eruption cysts Giant cell granuloma Kaposi sarcoma
Red	Angioma Carcinoma Giant cell granuloma Granulomatous disorders Kaposi sarcoma Pyogenic granuloma (Figure 25.4)
White	Carcinoma Papillomas Verrucous leukoplakia Warts
Yellow	Calculi Lipomas Osseous lesions (e.g. Tori) Lymphoepithelial cyst

Mucosal swellings may be seen in some hereditary conditions, reactive lesions (trauma, inflammatory conditions, angioedema), granulomatous conditions, infections, neoplasms, deposits (e.g. amyloidosis), other disorders and as a reaction to certain drugs (Table 25.1).

Swellings may be hard if related to calcified substances, firm if neoplastic or hyperplastic, soft in granulomatous conditions, or fluctuant in, for example, angioedema, angiomas, inflammatory edema or mucoceles and this helps differentiation (Figure 25.1). Swellings may be colored (Table 25.2).

Hereditary gingival fibromatosis (HGF)

Definition: Familial generalized gingival fibromatosis.

Prevalence (approximate): Uncommon; 1 in 9,000.

Age mainly affected: From childhood.

Gender mainly affected: M = F.

Etiopathogenesis: Autosomal dominant condition due to chromosome 2 or 5 anomalies, resulting in transforming growth factor stimulation of fibroblast proliferation with altered matrix metalloproteinase expression.

Diagnostic features

History

Oral: The family history is positive. Generalized painless gingival enlargement is obvious, especially during the transition from deciduous to permanent dentition.

Extraoral: Hirsutism.

Clinical features

Oral: The gingivae are enlarged, usually of normal colour but firm in consistency, and the surface, although initially smooth, becomes coarsely stippled (Figure 25.5). The enlargements initially involve the papillae and later the attached gingiva and if gross, may move or cover the teeth and bulge out of the mouth. There are occasional associations with supernumerary teeth.

Extraoral: There may be associations with hirsutism, epilepsy, sensorineural deafness and rare syndromes, such as Laband (with skeletal anomalies), Byars-Jurkiewicz (giant fibroadenomas), Rutherford (corneal dystrophy), Cowden (multiple hamartomas) and Cross (oculocerebral-hypopigmentation) syndromes.

Differential diagnosis: Drug-induced gingival swelling; juvenile hyaline fibromatosis and infantile systemic hyalinosis.

Investigations: Diagnosis is clinical. Microscopy shows grossly increased fibrous tissue which otherwise appears normal and usually elongation of the epithelial rete ridges – features identical to those in drug-associated gingival swelling. The gingival connective tissue is mainly composed of thick interlacing collagen fibres forming a dense, almost avascular mass in which many fibrocytes have dark shrunken nuclei. Mucoid material and some giant cells may be seen.

Management

Surgery often indicated.

Prognosis

Excellent. Recurrences may occur.

C1 esterase inhibitor deficiency (hereditary angioedema)

Most angioedema is allergic (Quincke edema), presenting with sudden painless, circumscribed, non-pitting swelling of face (around the eyes, chin, and lips), tongue, feet, genitalia, and trunk, which persists from hours to three days after allergen-exposure. Involvement of the upper airways can result in life-threatening symptoms, including the risk of asphyxiation, unless appropriate interventions are taken.

Hereditary angioedema (HAE) is an autosomal dominant disease that afflicts up to 1 in 10,000 persons and presents comparable risks. HAE patients often have C1-inhibitor (CI-INH) deficiency.

HAE attacks are triggered by trauma (especially dental), anxiety, menstruation, infection, exercise, alcohol, and stress, but attacks can occur in the absence of any identifiable initiating event. Medications (e.g. estrogens, angiotensin converting enzyme inhibitors, angiotensin II type 1 receptor antagonists) can also be triggers.

Attacks are mediated by vascular permeability enhancing factors generated via contact system activation, a system usually controlled by C1-INH. This is the major inhibitor of activated factor XII (Hageman factor) and kallikrein, the contact system protease that cleaves kininogen and releases bradykinin.

Analyses of C1 INH, C4 and C1q should be performed. Acute exacerbations of HAE should be treated with intravenous purified C1 esterase inhibitor concentrate.

Drug-induced gingival swelling

Gingival swelling (sometimes termed "hyperplasia") is a recognized adverse effect of hydantoins such as phenytoin (in around 50% of users), calcium-channel blockers (dihydropyridines, especially nifedipine, in around 25%) and ciclosporin (in around 25%). Valproate and estrogen have occasionally been associated with gingival overgrowth.

The gene encoding CTLA-4 (Cytotoxic T-lymphocyte antigen 4), a molecule influencing T cell activation may influence the gingival swelling. There is no correlation between the extent of overgrowth and the dose of drug, its serum level, or the age and gender of the patient. Rather, the swelling is aggravated by poor oral hygiene. The gingival enlargement characteristically affects the interdental papillae first but may later involve the marginal and even attached gingiva (Figure 25.6). The palatal and lingual gingivae are usually involved less than the buccal and labial gingivae. The enlargement is characteristically firm, pale and tough, with coarse stippling, although these features may take several years to develop, and earlier lesions may be softer and redder.

Management

The patient's level of plaque control should be improved and a 0.2% aqueous chlorhexidine mouthwash may be helpful. Excision of the enlarged tissue may be indicated.

Prognosis

Excellent. Recurrences may occur, although this is less likely with meticulous oral hygiene, particularly if the drug can be stopped.

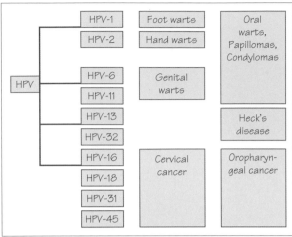

HPV-1	Foot warts	Oral warts, Papillomas, Condylomas
HPV-2	Hand warts	
HPV-6	Genital warts	
HPV-11		
HPV-13		Heck's disease
HPV-32		
HPV-16	Cervical cancer	Oropharyn-geal cancer
HPV-18		
HPV-31		
HPV-45		

Figure 26.1 HPV types and their associations.

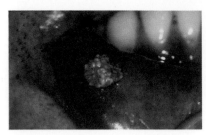

Figure 26.2 Papilloma.

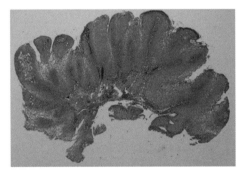

Figure 26.3 HPV papilloma.

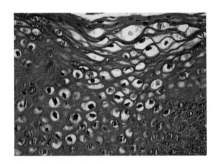

Figure 26.4 HPV koilocytes.

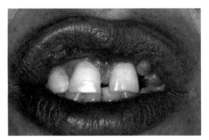

Figure 26.5 Oral warts.

The **H**uman **P**apilloma **V**irus (HPV) infection is contagious when there is contact with the skin or mucosa of an infected person. Transmitted usually by close contact, often in childhood, most cause benign epithelial growths (warts), though lesions may not always be clinically evident. Skin warts typically disappear after a few months but can last for years and the virus remains and can recur especially in people who are immunocompromised as in HIV/AIDS or transplant recipients. HPV infections can also occur in the mouth and can be transmitted by oral-oral or oro-anogenital contact.

There are over 100 strains of HPV (Figure 26.1). Types 1, 2, and 3 cause common skin warts: Type 1 causes warts on the soles of feet and palm of the hands. Type 2 causes common warts, filiform warts, plantar warts, and mosaic plantar warts. Type 3 causes "plane" or flat warts.

Types 6 and 11 cause anogenital warts. HPV types 16 and 18 cause about 70% of cervical cancer and are thus termed "high risk" types. A higher prevalence of HPV infections is seen in patients with other sexually transmitted infections.

Oral papillomas are far more common than warts or condylomas but the various forms of oral "warts" are clinically difficult to differentiate and have not always been typed.

Papilloma

Definition: A benign epithelial neoplasm with an anemone-like appearance.

Prevalence (approximate): Uncommon.

Age mainly affected: Adults.

Gender mainly affected: M = F.

Etiopathogenesis: HPV 6 or 11. Common in HIV-infected people and increased after therapy with ART.

Diagnostic features
Clinical features
Oral: A small, white or pink, cauliflower-like, sessile or pedunculated lesion, < 1 cm in diameter. Most common at the junction of the hard and soft palate; the lips (Figure 26.2), gingiva or tongue may occasionally be affected.

They appear to be, and remain, benign, unlike papillomas of the larynx or bowel, which may undergo malignant transformation.

Differential diagnosis: Other warty lesions; fibroepithelial polyps.

Biopsy/histopathology: A fibrovascular core and extensions of the fibrovascular core covered by acanthotic stratified squamous epithelium

(Figure 26.3). The epithelium shows no evidence of dysplasia but there may be some koilocytic change – clear cells with the nucleus pushed to one side (Figure 26.4), a feature of some viral infections.

Management
Papillomas are best removed and examined histologically to establish the diagnosis. Excision must be total, deep and wide enough to include any abnormal cells beyond the zone of the pedicle. Cryosurgery or pulse dye laser or carbon dioxide (CO_2) laser may be used.

Some use salicylic acid, imiquimod or topical podophyllum resin paint, but this is potentially teratogenic and toxic to brain, kidney and myocardium.

Prognosis
Good.

Warts (verrucae)
Definition: Verrucae are common skin warts; condylomata acuminatum are anogenital warts (venereal warts).

Prevalence (approximate): Uncommon.

Age mainly affected: Verrucae are usually seen on the lips of children who have warts on the fingers. Condylomata are usually seen on the tongue or fauces in sexually active adults.

Gender mainly affected: M = F.

Etiopathogenesis: Verrucae are usually caused by HPV 2, 4, 40, or 57. Condyloma acuminata are usually caused by HPV 6, 11, 16, or 18, are highly contagious and are sexually transmitted through direct skin-to-skin contact during oral, genital, or anal sex with an infected partner. In HIV disease, HPV 7, 72 or 73 may be found.

Diagnostic features
Clinical features
Oral: Verrucae are found predominantly on the lips (Figure 26.5); condyloma acuminata are found on the tongue, or palate. They can either be warty papules or more smooth-surfaced.

Differential diagnosis: Other warts; fibrocpithelial polyps.

Histopathological changes include acanthotic and sometimes hyperkeratotic epithelium with occasional koilocytosis.

Management
Excision, which must be total, deep and wide enough to include any abnormal cells beyond the zone of the pedicle. Cryosurgery or pulse dye laser or carbon dioxide (CO_2) laser may be used.

Salicylic acid, topical podophyllum resin paint, fluorouracil, imiquimod or intralesional alpha interferon may be effective.

Prognosis
Good. Recurrence may occur.

Multifocal epithelial hyperplasia (Heck disease)
This is a rare, benign, familial disorder characterized by multiple, soft, circumscribed, sessile, nodular elevations of the oral mucosa. Seen particularly in native Americans and in Inuits in Greenland, where the prevalence approaches 35%, it has been reported rarely from many other countries. HPV-13 and HPV-32 appear to be causal in patients with genetic predisposition to the disease.

Among native Americans, multifocal epithelial hyperplasia mainly affects children and usually involves the lower lip, cheeks and tongue, whereas in the Inuit and in white people the lesions are found mainly in the fourth decade and later and often affect the tongue and lips.

The characteristics of multifocal epithelial hyperplasia are acanthosis with broad, elongated and often fused rete ridges. Epithelial cells of the intermediate layer may have a pseudomitotic appearance.

This is a benign asymptomatic condition, requiring only reassurance. Surgical excision is indicated in traumatized (hyperplastic) lesions and in persistent cases producing esthetic or functional alterations.

Koilocytic dysplasia
This is a pathological description of a papillomavirus-associated lesion that presents as a white flat or elevated lesion seen in the lingual, buccal or labial mucosa, sometimes in HIV-infected individuals. HPV 6/11, 16/18, or 31/33/51 are implicated; the prognosis is uncertain but there are some features of dysplasia.

HPV and oral cancer
HPV16 is frequently associated with oropharyngeal carcinoma. Whether the HPV vaccine now being given to young people to prevent anogenital infections and cervical cancer will protect against mouth cancer, remains to be seen.

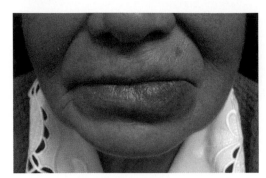

Figure 27.1a *Granulomatous cheilitis (Melkersson-Rosenthal syndrome).*

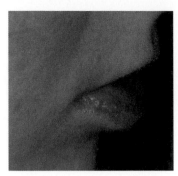

Figure 27.1b *Granulomatous cheilitis (Melkersson-Rosenthal syndrome).*

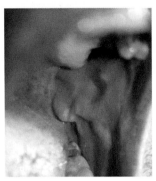

Figure 27.2 *Cobblestone pattern in Crohn disease.*

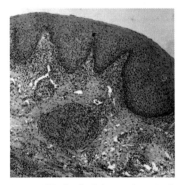

Figure 27.3 *Orofacial granulomatosis.*

A *granuloma* is an organized collection of macrophages, with lymphocytes, giant cells and fibrosis, sometimes necrosis, which arises as a reaction to an antigen.

The term "granulomatous" refers to inflammatory diseases or reactions characterized by granulomas. In the mouth, these include:
- *Granulomatous reactions to:*
  — *unknown antigens* (e.g. sarcoidosis, Crohn disease and orofacial granulomatosis (OFG))
  — *foreign bodies* (e.g. to silicone used as esthetic filler in lips)
  — *infections* (e.g. tuberculosis and mycoses)
- *Wegener granulomatosis* – a granulomatous reaction with necrotizing vasculitis, and infiltrating neutrophils, eosinophils and lymphocytes.

The term granuloma is also used in oral lesions such as pyogenic granuloma, giant cell granuloma and periapical granuloma but is then inappropriate, since none are granulomatous reactions.

Sarcoidosis

This presents with cervical lymphadenopathy, enlarged salivary glands and xerostomia. Heerfordt syndrome (salivary and lacrimal swelling, facial palsy and uveitis), mucosal nodules, gingival or labial swelling are rare. Diagnosis is by biopsy (minor salivary gland biopsy reveals granulomas in 20%), chest radiography, gallium scan, raised serum angiotensin converting enzyme (SACE) and adenosine deaminase.

Management is with intralesional corticosteroids; systemic corticosteroids if lung or eye are involved.

Crohn disease and orofacial granulomatosis

This is a chronic inflammatory bowel disease that affects mainly the ileum, but it can affect any part of the gastrointestinal tract including the mouth (OFG is similar but appears to affect only the mouth).

Prevalence (approximate): Uncommon.

Age mainly affected: From childhood; usually second and third decades.

Gender mainly affected: M > F.

Etiopathogenesis: Crohn disease is of unknown cause. Jewish ancestry is a risk factor. With a bimodal age distribution of disease onset with peaks at 20 and 50 years, evidence suggests it may represent an abnormal mucosal T-lymphocyte response to commensal bacteria in genetically predisposed individuals. The inflammatory response is mediated by factors such as tumor necrosis factor (TNF) alpha. Implicated are the CARD15 gene and perhaps *Mycobacterium paratuberculosis* infection.

Patients diagnosed with OFG develop similar oral lesions, and probably have a latent, limited or precursor form of Crohn disease. Sometimes, OFG develops because of an adverse reaction to food additives, such as cinnamaldehyde, tartrazine or benzoates, butylated hydroxyanisole or dodecyl gallate (in margarine), or to menthol (in peppermint oil) or cobalt.

Diagnostic features

History
Oral: Facial and/or labial swelling.

Extraoral: Crohn disease may present with abdominal pain, persistent diarrhea with passage of blood and mucus, anemia, and weight loss – all absent in OFG.

Clinical features
Oral features of Crohn disease and OFG may include, in any combination:
- facial and/or labial swelling (Figure 27.1a and b) (Miescher or granulomatous cheilitis is a term used when this is the only lesion evident); Melkersson-Rosenthal syndrome is where lip or facial swelling is seen with fissured tongue and facial palsy (in 30% of cases)
- angular stomatitis and/or cracked lips
- ulcers
- mucosal tags and/or cobble stoning (Figure 27.2)
- gingival swelling.

Oral lesions in Crohn disease are most likely in those who develop skin, eye or joint complications.

Extraoral: Abdominal pain, persistent diarrhea with passage of blood and mucus, anemia, and weight loss.

Differential diagnosis: Local infections; angioedema; sarcoidosis; Ascher syndrome (lip swelling associated with blepharochalasia and goitre present from childhood).

Blood investigations, including full blood picture, and levels of albumin, calcium, folate, iron and vitamin B12 may reveal malabsorption. Imaging intestinal radiology (barium enema), sigmoidoscopy and colonoscopy, and biopsy may reveal gastrointestinal Crohn lesions but, as the lesions may be scattered, a negative result cannot necessarily exclude the condition. An oral biopsy may confirm the presence of lymphedema and granulomas, but cannot reliably differentiate Crohn disease from OFG or sarcoidosis. Biopsy during the early stages shows only edema and perivascular lymphocytic infiltration. In some cases of long duration no other changes are seen, but in others the infiltrate becomes more dense and pleomorphic and small focal granulomas are seen. The most obvious feature is that in the papillary corium there is pronounced edema, in some areas there is fibrin exudation and dilatation of the superficial lymphatics. In other areas there is a patchy chronic inflammatory cell infiltration (which is predominantly lymphocytic and to a lesser extent plasmacytic). Most of these changes are in the superficial part of the lesion, but may extend deeply into muscle. Granulomas are usually poorly formed, with an indiscrete edge and without a well-defined lymphocytic cuff around them or fibrosis (Figure 27.3). Also, multinucleated giant cells are often scattered or absent. The granulomas can sometimes bulge into, or occasionally lie free in the lymphatics, which they may block (endovasal granulomatous lymphangitis), producing the edema which is presumably responsible for the swellings.

Dietary-related cases of OFG can only be confirmed by an exclusion diet to eliminate food allergens. Skin tests may be useful to reveal various likely reactants. Sarcoidosis may need to be excluded.

Management
Crohn disease should be treated by a physician. Secondary deficiencies should be corrected. In OFG, an exclusion diet should be tried (cinnamon and/or benzoate-free diets). Intralesional corticosteroids may help control lesions such as swelling, and occasionally systemic sulfasalazine or other agents (clofazimine, metronidazole, ketotifen, infliximab or thalidomide) are required.

In some circumstances, resection of areas of intestinal lesions is indicated.

Prognosis
Some patients with OFG have latent systemic disease, especially Crohn disease, which develops months or years later, but others appear to remain otherwise healthy. Some people have long remissions. Regular follow-up should ensure that systemic disease is recognized early.

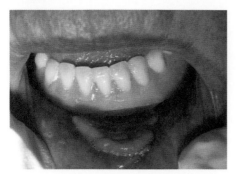

Figure 28.1 Denture induced hyperplasia.

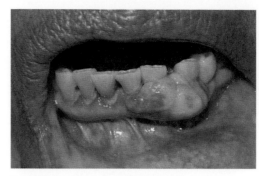

Figure 28.2 Inflammatory fibrous epulis.

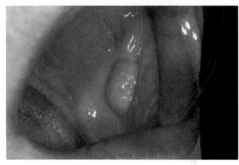

Figure 28.3 Fibrous lump.

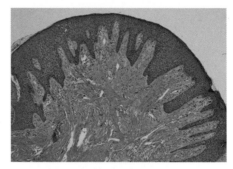

Figure 28.4 Fibrous hyperplasia.

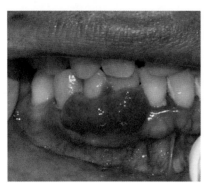

Figure 28.5 Pyogenic granuloma.

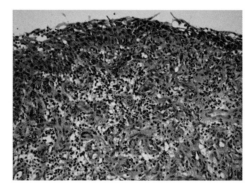

Figure 28.6 Pyogenic granuloma.

Denture-induced hyperplasia (epulis fissuratum)

Definition: Hyperplasia related to an overextended denture flange.

Prevalence (approximate): Common.

Age mainly affected: Middle-aged or older patients.

Gender mainly affected: F > M.

Etiopathogenesis: Where a denture flange irritates the vestibular mucosa, an ulcer and then a linear reparative process may be initiated. In time, an elongated fibroepithelial enlargement may develop. Such a lesion (once called a denture granuloma) is little different in structure from a fibroepithelial polyp.

Diagnostic features

History

Oral: Usually a symptomless lump.

Clinical features

Oral: Usually related to ill-fitting lower complete denture, especially anteriorly. Typically a lump with a smooth pink surface lying parallel with the alveolar ridge and sometimes grooved or ulcerated by the denture flange (Figure 28.1). Several leaflets with a fairly firm consistency may develop.

Differential diagnosis: fibrous lumps and neoplasms.

Management

Relieve the denture flange but, if this does not induce the lesion to regress within two to three weeks, the lump should be excised and examined histologically.

Prognosis

Good.

Fibroepithelial polyp (fibrous lump)

Fibrous lumps should not be confused with the true fibroma, a benign neoplasm derived from fibroblasts, which is rare in the mouth (see below). Fibrous lumps are common in the mouth, seen mainly in adults and appear to be purely reparative in nature following trauma or irritation (e.g. biting).

Fibrous lumps vary from red, shiny, soft lumps to those which are pale, stippled and firm. Commonly, they are painless, round pedunculated swellings arising from the marginal or papillary gingiva (epulides) (Figure 28.2), tongue, or buccal mucosa (Figure 28.3) or lips (often at the occlusal line – presumably induced by trauma). Typically the epithelium is either normal or hyperplastic, beneath which is an area of fibroblastic proliferation and collagenisation, sometimes with heavy inflammation. The bulk of the lesion consists of a vascular stroma with plump fibroblasts with large vesicular nuclei and prominent nucleoli (Figure 28.4). There may be mitotic activity which can be somewhat alarming at higher power. Dystrophic calcification where calcium salts have been deposited around non-vital tissue is common in fibrous epulides and there also tends to be osseous metaplasia.

Fibrous epulides should be removed down to the periosteum, which should be curetted thoroughly.

Fibroma

Fibroma is a benign neoplasm of fibroblastic origin, rare in the oral cavity. It presents as a continuously enlarging pedunculated growth with a smooth, non-ulcerated, pink surface, most often located on the buccal mucosa along the plane of occlusion. Differential diagnosis includes neurofibroma, peripheral giant cell granuloma, mucocele, and salivary gland tumors. The fibroma should be totally excised; histology shows marked proliferation of fibroblasts, with nuclei of uniform shape, size and staining characteristics. Recurrence is possible.

Giant cell epulis (peripheral giant cell granuloma)

The giant cell epulis probably arises because chronic irritation triggers a reactionary hyperplasia of mucoperiosteum and excessive production of granulation tissue. Most patients are in the fourth to sixth decades. A slight female predilection has been described. Classically, it is a swelling with a deep-red color (although older lesions tend to be paler) that often arises interdentally, but only anterior to the permanent molars.

Although a benign lesion it should be excised. Histologically there is usually a cell-free zone between the main lesion and the overlying epithelium but this zone tends to be lost if there has been inflammation or ulceration. There is a matrix or stroma of plump spindle-shaped cells in which there are multinucleated giant cells. These are sometimes so confluent that it can be difficult to see the outlines of the cells. They are large and contain about 10–20 nuclei. The giant cell epulis can be extremely vascular and sometimes the multinucleated giant cells are seen within vascular spaces. There may be considerable amounts of hemosiderin in these lesions. Mitotic activity is usually not difficult to find, but bears no relation to the clinical behavior. Osseous metaplasia is common and sometimes florid. Giant cell epulides tend to recur.

Pyogenic granuloma

Pyogenic granuloma commonly affects the gingiva (Figure 28.5), the lip or the tongue. It may be caused by chronic irritation and appears predisposed in patients who have had organ transplantation. It is clinically identical to peripheral giant cell granuloma and peripheral ossifying fibroma. Histopathologically there are many anastomosing vascular channels, usually with plump endothelial cell nuclei (Figure 28.6). The vessels often show a clustered or medullary pattern, leading some authorities to consider it as a polypoid form of capillary hemangioma or an inflamed lobular hemangioma. The stroma is edematous, but older lesions may have fibrosed. Chronic and acute inflammatory cells are scattered throughout the stroma, with early lesions containing more neutrophils.

The lesion should be excised completely but will readily recur if excision is inadequate.

Pregnancy epulis is a pyogenic granuloma arising as an exaggerated inflammatory reaction to dental bacterial plaque in pregnancy (prevalence 1%). Oral hygiene should be improved. Most lesions tend to resolve on parturition. A pregnancy epulis requires excision only if it is being traumatized or is grossly unesthetic.

Peripheral Ossifying Fibroma (POF)

The gingiva is a common site of fibrous inflammatory hyperplasia, that clinically can be similar to pyogenic granuloma, peripheral giant cell granuloma and peripheral ossifying fibroma. The latter is a reactive growth due trauma or local irritants and should not be considered as the counterpart of the more aggressive central ossifying fibroma. POF occurs only in the gingiva and microscopically is characterized by bone and cement like calcifications in a fibrous stroma formed by spindle cells probably derived from the periodont ligament. Usually areas of gingival inflammation and vascular hyperplasia similar to pyogenic granuloma are present. If only dystrophic calcification and inflammation is seen, the diagnosis is of gingival inflammatory hyperplasia. Treatment is surgical, but recurrences can occur.

Swellings: Malignant neoplasms, oral squamous cell carcinoma (OSCC)

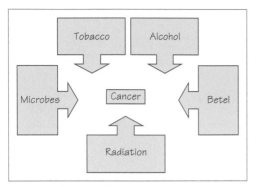

Figure 29.1 OSCC risk factors.

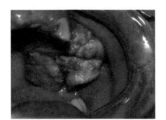

Figure 29.2 OSCC etiopathogenesis.

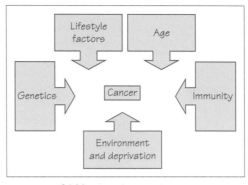

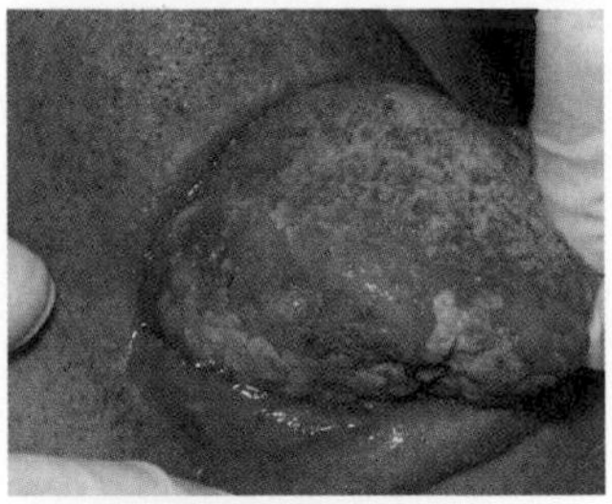

Figure 29.3a Squamous cell carcinoma.

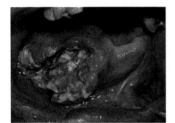

Figure 29.3b Squamous cell carcinoma.

Figure 29.3c Squamous cell carcinoma.

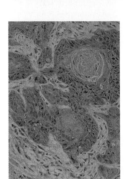

Figure 29.4 Squamous carcinoma biopsy/histopathology .

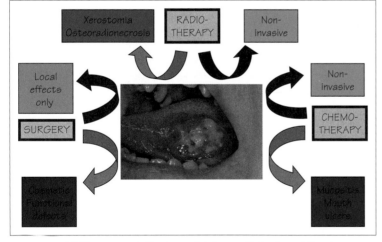

Figure 29.5 OSCC treatment. Courtesy of J. Bagan, C. Scully and Elsevier.

Table 29.1 TNM classification of malignant neoplasms.

Primary tumor size (T)	Comment
Tx	No available information
T0	No evidence of primary tumor
Tis	Carcinoma in situ
T1–T4	T1, 2 cm maximum diameter; T2, 2–4 cm; T3, > 4 cm; T4 > 4 cm, with involvement of adjacent structures
Regional lymph node involvement (N)	
Nx	Nodes not assessed
N0	No clinically positive nodes
N1	Single ipsilateral node < 3 cm
N2a	Single ipsilateral nodes 3–6 cm
N2b	Multiple ipsilateral nodes < 6 cm
N2c	Bilateral or contralateral nodes < 6 cm
N3	Any node > 6 cm
Distant metastases (M)	
Mx	Not assessed
M0	No evidence
M1	Present

Definition: Oral squamous cell carcinoma (OSCC) is a malignant neoplasm of stratified squamous epithelium.

Prevalence (approximate): The eighth most common cancer worldwide. Northern France, Eastern Europe, South America and South East Asia have high prevalences. Prevalence is rising in many countries.

Age mainly affected: Middle-aged and older, though younger people seem increasingly at risk.

Gender mainly affected: M > F.

Etiopathogenesis: Risk factors include especially tobacco and alcohol (Figure 29.1). The combination of heavy smoking and alcohol abuse is synergistic. Betel chewing, radiation, and infections may be implicated, and age, genetics, immune competence and diet, especially low fruit and vegetable consumption, are also relevant (Figure 29.2). Infections such as candidosis and syphilis have been implicated, and human papillomavirus (HPV, mainly HPV-16) has been implicated in oropharyngeal carcinoma.

DNA mutations affect genes, particularly oncogenes (e.g. epidermal growth factor receptor; EGFR) whose over-activity then drives cell proliferation. In contrast, tumor suppressor gene (TSG) mutations or deletions inhibit activity of TSGs such as p16 (checkpoints in growth control) and p53 (which either repairs a potentially malignant cell or destroys it by apoptosis). Cells thus become able to proliferate uncontrollably (autonomously) and cancer results, characterized by invasion across the epithelial basement membrane and, ultimately, metastasis to lymph nodes, bone, brain, liver and other sites.

Liver carcinogen metabolizing enzymes protect by degrading carcinogens. DNA repair enzymes and may repair mutations.

Second primary neoplasms are seen in up to 25% over three years, and in up to 40% of those who continue to smoke tobacco.

Potentially malignant disorders include some:
- erythroplakia
- leukoplakia
- lichen planus
- oral submucous fibrosis
- immunosuppression
- tertiary syphilis
- discoid lupus erythematosus
- dyskeratosis congenita
- Paterson-Kelly syndrome (sideropenic dysphagia).

Diagnostic features
History
Oral: Typically up to six months delay before diagnosis, as pain is not an early feature.

Clinical features
Oral: Any solitary lump, ulcer, white or red lesion persisting for more than three weeks or non-healing socket, numbness, or unexplained loose tooth is suspect as OSCC until proven otherwise (Figures 29.3a–c).

Lip carcinoma typically presents at the vermilion border of the lower lip; intraoral carcinoma typically affects the postero-lateral tongue/floor of mouth.

Synchronous and metachronous second primary tumors (SPTs) may appear elsewhere in the oral cavity.

Extraoral: Cervical lymphadenopathy may be detectable. SPTs may be found in the upper aerodigestive tract (pharynx, larynx, esophagus).

Differential diagnosis: Lip carcinoma from herpes labialis, keratoacanthoma, and basal cell carcinoma. Intraoral carcinoma from aphthae, other neoplasms or chronic infections.

It is crucial to determine the diagnosis, extent of spread, whether cervical lymph nodes are involved or if there are other primary tumors, or metastases elsewhere. SPTs must be excluded by imaging, endoscopy and biopsy.

Oral lesional biopsy/histopathology is indicated (Figure 29.4). In well-differentiated OSCC the epithelium forms islands invading the underlying tissues and undergoing aberrant keratinisation. Keratin forms within epithelial islands producing whorls or epithelial pearls, instead of being shed from the surface. Moderately differentiated OSCC consists of small epithelial islands with a high mitotic index, nuclear hyperchromatism but no obvious keratinization. Poorly differentiated OSCC contains sheets of cells showing extreme pleomorphism, giant nuclei and multiple and bizarre mitoses.

Potential imaging techniques to detect residual and recurrent locoregional disease after treatment are (serial) CT or MRI and FDG-PET (Positron Emission Tomography (PET) scanning).

Management
OSCC is usually staged using the TNM (Tumor Node Metastasis) system (Table 29.1).

Management is guided especially by the balance between positive outcomes and adverse effects but is largely by surgery, with radiotherapy or sometimes chemotherapy (Figure 29.5).

The tumor is ideally resected with a 2 cm margin, to remove all tissue with malignant potential. Free tissue transfer (tissue with its own arterial supply and venous drainage) is used to replace ablated tissue. Metastases, when present, occur in cervical lymph nodes in almost 80%, and their removal (lymphadenectomy) by selective neck dissection is indicated.

Radiotherapy (RT) has a role in management of early and locally advanced OSCC alone or, more frequently with surgery and/or increasingly chemotherapy. Attempts to improve RT efficacy while maintaining acceptable toxicities (mucositis, dry mouth, trismus, osteoradionecrosis), include Intensity Modulated RadioTherapy (IMRT), Image Guided Radiation Therapy (IGRT) and Concomitant Chemo-radiotherapy (CT-RT).

TPF (Taxanes, Platinum (cisplatin) and 5-Fluorouracil) is the standard chemotherapy regimen. Cetuximab (anti-EGFR), if added, produces a survival benefit.

Persons with carcinoma must be advised to stop any tobacco/alcohol/betel habits, and encouraged to have a diet rich in fruit and vegetables.

Prognosis
Prognosis is best in early well-differentiated and not metastasized OSCC, but depends mainly on tumor size, completeness of resection, and nodal involvement. The prognosis of intraoral carcinoma is about a 30–50% five-year survival rate because of the high proportion of late stage cases. Lip cancer, typically detected earlier, has a better survival, often > 70% five-year survival.

30 Swellings: Malignant neoplasms, lymphoma, metastatic neoplasms

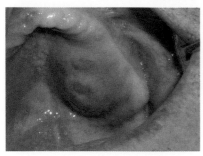

Figure 30.1 Lymphoma.

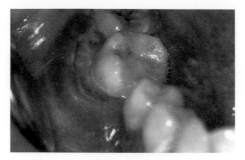

Figure 30.2 Lymphoma (from Bagan JV, Scully C. Medicina y Patologia Oral, 2006).

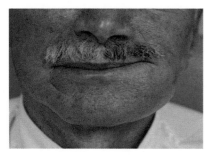

Figure 30.3a Non-Hodgkin lymphoma.

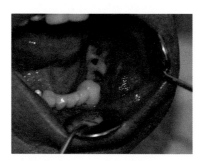

Figure 30.3b Non-Hodgkin lymphoma.

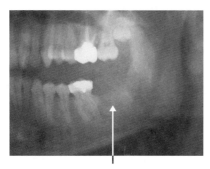

Figure 30.3c Non-Hodgkin lymphoma.

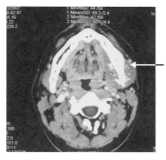

Figure 30.3d Non-Hodgkin lymphoma.

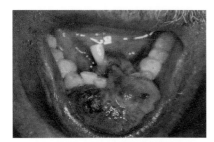

Figure 30.4 Metastasis of carcinoma.

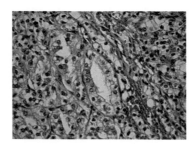

Figure 30.5 Metastasis of renal cell carcinoma.

Lymphomas

Definition: Malignant neoplasm arising from lymphocytes; based on the "Revised European-American Lymphoma classification" (REAL), the WHO (2001, updated 2008) classified lymphomas in three broad groups (B, T or NK (natural killer)) according to cell type, plus less common groups e.g. Hodgkin lymphoma (HL).

Prevalence (approximate): Lymphomas are rare but, with the increase in HIV disease, are becoming more common.

Age mainly affected: Young adults. However, African Burkitt lymphoma typically affects children < 12–13 years age.

Gender mainly affected: M > F.

Etiopathogenesis: Lymphomas affecting the oral cavity are mainly B-cell lymphomas. Non-Hodgkin lymphoma (NHL) is more common in immunosuppression/HIV and autoimmune disease and often associated with Epstein-Barr virus (EBV; human herpesvirus-4). Plasmablastic lymphoma (polymorphic immunoblastic B lymphoproliferative disease) is predisposed by HIV disease and may be EBV-related, as is African Burkitt lymphoma (BL).

HL affects males predominantly and may have a family history, history of EBV infection, or rarely HIV or the prolonged use of growth hormone.

T-cell/NK angiocentric lymphomas (lethal midline granuloma) are related to EBV while T-cell lymphomas are occasionally associated with HTLV-1.

Diagnostic features

History
Oral: A lump or ulcer or loose teeth.

Extraoral: Night sweats, fatigue, weight loss, rashes, pruritus, painless enlargement of lymph nodes, pain following alcohol consumption, back pain.

Clinical features
Between 2–10% of lymphomas present first in the oral cavity and, of these, 80% are composed of follicular centre cells or post-follicular cells. Lymphomas usually affect the pharynx or palate, but occasionally the tongue, gingivae or lips; they may appear as swellings, which sometimes ulcerate and cause pain or sensory disturbance.

Oral: HL is rare and presents with enlarged rubbery lymph nodes, often in the neck, fever, pruritus, weight loss and night sweats and in advanced disease also with hepatosplenomegaly. NHL is more common, presents similarly but may be extra-nodal and then presents with lumps (Figure 30.1) or more usually non-healing painless ulcers (Figure 30.2), especially in the fauces, palate or maxillary gingivae, or with bony deposits, resulting in pain, anesthesia, swelling, tooth loosening, or pathological fracture. Polymorphic immunoblastic B lymphoproliferative disease presents as diffuse lumps or nodules, especially in the fauces or gingiva.

African BL commonly affects the jaws with massive swelling, which ulcerates into the mouth, pain, paresthesia or increasing tooth mobility. Discrete radiolucencies in the lower third molar region, destruction of lamina dura and widening of the periodontal space or teeth, which may appear to be "floating in air", may be radiographic features.

Extraoral: Fever, pruritus, weight loss and night sweats and in advanced disease also hepatosplenomegaly. Infections and other neoplasms are commonly associated.

Differential diagnosis: lymph node involvement mimics reactive immunoblastic processes (e.g. mononucleosis) and infections (e.g. Kikuchi lymphadenitis).

CT scanning with PET, or gallium scan, are used to detect small deposits (Figures 30.3a–d).

Biopsy/histopathology are mandatory. Lymphomas should be classified by histopathology and immunochemistry, and staged for the most appropriate therapy and prognostication, since some forms are indolent and compatible with a long life even without treatment, whereas other forms are aggressive.

Blood tests are performed to assess function of major organs, and erythrocyte sedimentation rate (ESR) which helps prognosis.

Staging (Ann Arbor classification):

Stage I – involvement of a single lymph node region (I) or single extralymphatic site (Ie)

Stage II – involvement of two or more lymph node regions on the same side of the diaphragm (II) or of one lymph node region and a contiguous extralymphatic site (IIe)

Stage III – involvement of lymph node regions on both sides of the diaphragm, which may include the spleen (IIIs) and/or limited contiguous extralymphatic organ or site (IIIe, IIIes)

Stage IV – disseminated involvement of one or more extralymphatic organs.

The absence of systemic symptoms is signified by adding "A" to the stage; the presence of systemic symptoms is noted by adding "B" to the stage. For localized extranodal extension from mass of nodes which does not advance the stage, subscript "E" is added.

Management
HL early stage disease (IA or IIA) is treated with radiotherapy or chemotherapy. Patients with later disease (III, IVA, or IVB) are treated with combination chemotherapy alone.

NHL is treated by combinations of radiotherapy or chemotherapy, monoclonal antibodies, immunotherapy and hematological stem cell transplantation.

Prognosis
HL has a 90% five-year survival; NHL has < 50% five-year survival.

Metastatic oral neoplasms

Metastases to the oral tissues are rare, accounting for only 1% of all oral tumors and most appear in bone, especially the mandibular premolar or molar area or condyle. Most metastases originate from carcinomas of breast, lung, kidney, thyroid, stomach, liver, colon, bone or prostate. Tumor deposits arise from lymphatic or hematogenous spread.

Metastases usually present as a lesion arising in the jaw, sometimes only revealed coincidentally by imaging, at other times causing symptoms. In up to one-third of patients the jaw lesions are the first manifestation of the tumor. Many metastases are asymptomatic but others manifest with:
- pain
- paresthesia or hypoesthesia
- swelling (Figure 30.4)
- tooth mobility
- non-healing extraction sockets
- pathological fracture
- radiolucency or radiopacity.

Diagnosis is from history and clinical features supplemented by imaging and histopathology (Figure 30.5).

Treatment is with radiotherapy, surgery or chemotherapy.

The prognosis is grave; the time from diagnosis of the metastasis to death is often only months.

31 Ulcers and erosions: Local causes, drug-induced ulcers

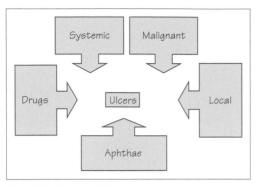

Figure 31.1 *Causes of ulcers.*

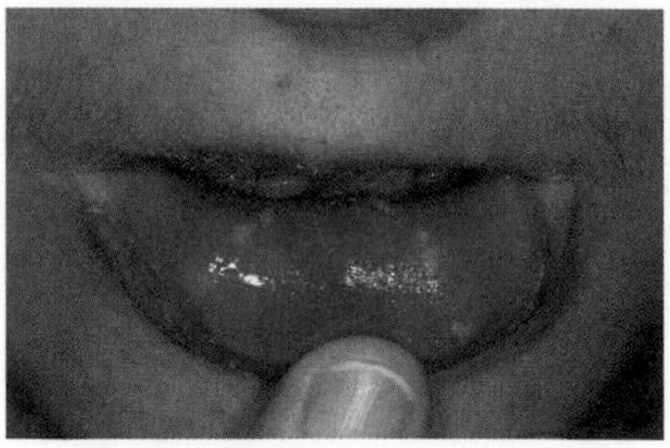

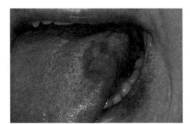

Figure 31.2 *Ulceration after biting the lip in a convulsion.*

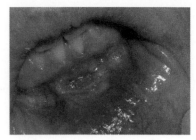

Figure 31.3 *Traumatic ulcer.*

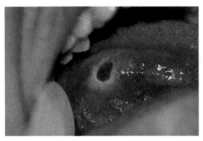

Figure 31.4 *Chronic traumatic ulcer.*

Figure 31.5 *Nicorandil-induced ulcer.*

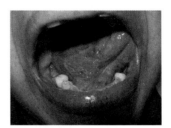

Figure 31.6 *Methotrexate-induced ulceration.*

Various infections or other systemic disorders, particularly those of blood, gastrointestinal tract or skin can produce mouth ulcers. Malignant neoplasms usually begin as swellings or lumps but may present as an ulcer. Mouth ulcers are often caused by trauma or burns, or aphthae, sometimes by drugs.

A useful mnemonic is **So Many Laws And Directives** (Figure 31.1) (Table 31.1).

Features that may aid diagnosis are ulcer numbers, shape, size, site, base, associated erythema, margin, and pain. A single ulcer, especially if persisting for three or more weeks is usually indicative of a chronic problem such as malignant disease or serious infection (e.g. tuberculosis or a fungal infection).

Local causes

Oral ulceration due to local factors is common. The history is typically of a single ulcer of short duration (5–10 days) with an obvious cause. Trauma may cause ulceration – typically of the lateral tongue, or the lip or buccal mucosa at the occlusal plane (Figure 31.2). Accidental cheek biting of an anesthetized lower lip or tongue following a dental local analgesic injection is fairly common in young children and those with learning disability. Orthodontic appliances or, more commonly, dentures (especially if new) are responsible for many traumatic ulcers and have been a problem in cleft-palate patients. Riga-Fede disease consists of ulcers of the lingual frenum in neonates with natal lower incisors, but similar ulcers may occur at other ages from coughing or cunnilingus. Oral purpura or ulceration may be seen on the palate in fellatio. The possibility of some other etiology for ulcers should always be borne in mind; child abuse may cause ulcers, especially over the upper labial frena.

Self-mutilation may be seen in patients who have psychological problems (Figure 31.3), learning or sensory impairment, or Lesch-

Nyhan syndrome. Chronic trauma may cause a well-defined ulcer with a whitish keratotic halo (Figure 31.4); the differential diagnosis may then include a neoplasm, lichen planus or lupus erythematosus.

Thermal burns, especially of the tongue and palate (e.g. "pizza burn" – now more common with microwave oven use), chemical burns, and irradiation mucositis may be seen.

Ulcers of local cause usually heal spontaneously within 7–14 days if the cause is removed. Maintenance of good oral hygiene and the use of hot saline mouthbaths and 0.2% aqueous chlorhexidine gluconate mouthwash aid healing. A 0.1% benzydamine mouthwash may help give relief. Occasionally, particularly in self-induced trauma, mechanical protection with a plastic guard may help.

Patients should be reviewed within three weeks to ensure healing has occurred. Any patient with a single ulcer lasting more than 2–3 weeks should be regarded with suspicion and investigated further; biopsy may be indicated.

Eosinophilic ulcer (traumatic eosinophilic granuloma; traumatic ulcerative granulomatous disease)

Eosinophilic ulcer is a rare, self-limiting ulcer that often appears on the tongue in children or older adults. The etiology remains obscure, but it may be associated with trauma, though drug reaction or an allergic response have also been suggested. Histopathological features include an extensive inflammatory cell infiltration with many eosinophilic cells throughout the submucosa and histological similarities to CD30+ T-lymphoproliferative disorders. The peripheral blood eosinophil count, however, is normal. Diagnosis and treatment is with either conservative excision or incisional biopsy.

Drug-induced ulcers (stomatitis medicamentosa)

A wide range of drugs can occasionally induce mouth ulcers, by a variety of effects. In some, there may also be lesions on skin or other mucosae. Drugs particularly implicated include:

- antianginal drugs such as nicorandil (Figure 31.5)
- antibiotics (metronidazole, penicillin, erythromycin, tetracycline)
- anticonvulsants (clonazepam, hydantoins, lamotrigine)
- antidepressants (imipramine, fluoxetine)
- antihypertensives (captopril, enalapril, propranolol)
- anti-inflammatory agents such as NSAIDs (aspirin, ibuprofen, indometacin, naproxen)
- antimalarials (chloroquine)
- antimitotic drugs used in chemotherapy (Figure 31.6) (cisplatin, ciclosporin, doxorubicin, methotrexate, vincristine)
- antiretrovirals (ritonavir, saquinavir, zidovudine).

Oral use of caustics or agents such as cocaine can cause erosions or ulcers. Chemical burns due, for example, to holding mouthwashes in the mouth or drugs against the buccal mucosa, can cause white sloughing lesions. Suggested associations of oral LP with systemic disease such as diabetes mellitus and hypertension (Grinspan syndrome) are most probably explained by drug-induced lichenoid lesions (Chapter 39). Erythema multiforme and toxic epidermal necrolysis (Chapter 36) may be drug-induced. Pemphigoid can be induced by penicillamine and furosemide. Pemphigus can be induced by captopril and other drugs (mercaptopropionyl glycine, penicillamine, penicillins, piroxicam, pyritinol, rifampicin, 5 thiopyridoxine, tiopronine).

Diagnosis is made from the drug history and testing the effect of withdrawal. Skin patch tests are rarely of practical value.

Ulcers caused by drugs usually resolve in 10–14 days if the offending drug can be identified and withdrawn. Treat ulceration symptomatically with topical benzydamine and possibly chlorhexidine.

Table 31.1 Causes of oral ulceration.

Systemic		Malignant	Local	Aphthae	Drugs & others
Blood	Anemia Sideropenia Hypoplasminogenemia Neutropenias Leukemias Myelofibrosis Myelodysplasia Multiple myeloma Giant-cell arteritis Periarteritis nodosa	Carcinoma and other malignant tumors Langerhans cell histiocytoses Wegener granulomatosis	Burns (chemical, electrical, thermal, radiation) Trauma (may be artifactual)	Recurrent aphthous stomatitis	Drugs: Cytotoxics, NSAIDs, nicorandil, many others
Infections	Aspergillosis Atypical mycobacterial infections Blastomycosis Coccidioidomycosis Cryptococcosis Cytomegalovirus infection Gram-negative bacteria Hand, foot and mouth disease Herpangina Herpes simplex Histoplasmosis HIV infection Infectious mononucleosis Leishmaniasis Lepromatous leprosy Mucormycosis Necrotising ulcerative gingivitis Paracoccidioidomycosis Syphilis Tuberculosis Tularemia Varicella-zoster			Aphthous-like ulcers (including Behçet syndrome/MAGIC syndrome, Sweet syndrome and acute febrile illness of childhood (PFAPA: Periodic fever, aphthae, pharyngitis, adenitis))	Other conditions: Angiolymphoid hyperplasia with eosinophilia, hypereosinophilic syndrome, necrotizing sialometaplasia
Gastrointestinal	Celiac disease Crohn disease Orofacial granulomatosis Ulcerative colitis				
Skin and connective tissue	Dermatitis herpetiformis Epidermolysis bullosa Epidermolysis bullosa acquisita Chronic ulcerative stomatitis Graft-versus-host disease Erythema multiforme Lichen planus Linear IgA disease Pemphigoid Pemphigus Felty syndrome Lupus erythematosus Mixed connective tissue disease Reiter disease				

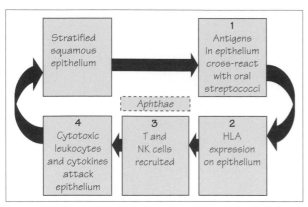
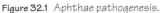

Figure 32.1 Aphthae pathogenesis.

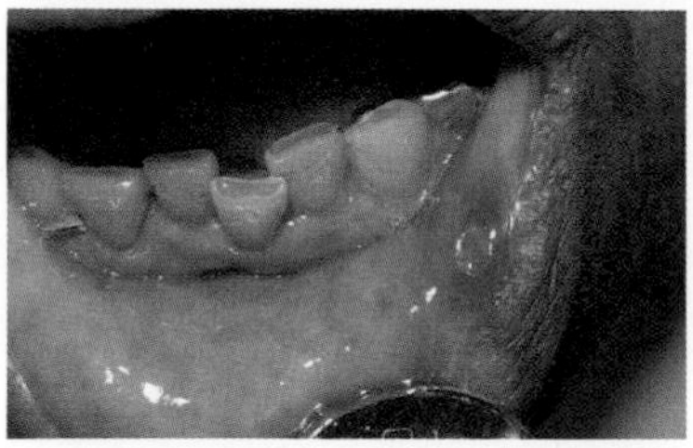

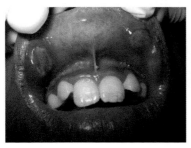

Figure 32.2 Recurrent aphthous stomatis (RAS) minor.

Figure 32.3 RAS major.

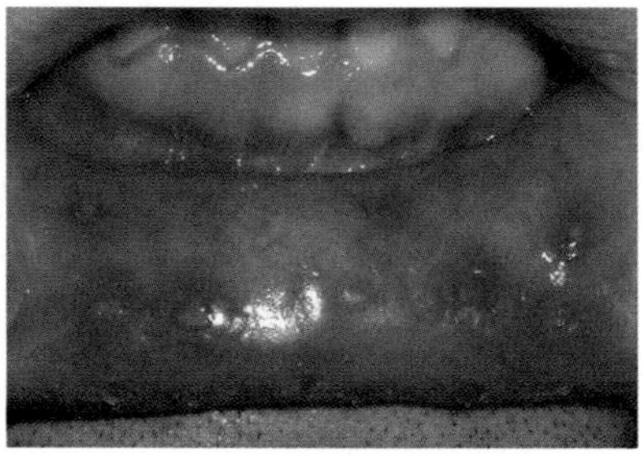

Figure 32.4 RAS herpetiform ulcers.

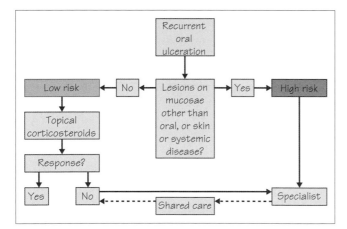

Figure 32.5 Recurrent oral ulcers: management.

Definition: Aphthae are recurrent mouth ulcers which typically start in childhood, have a natural history to improve with age and are unassociated with systemic disease.

Prevalence (approximate): 25–60% of the population.

Age mainly affected: Children and young adults.

Gender mainly affected: F > M.

Etiopathogenesis: There may be a family history and weak HLA associations suggesting a genetic predisposition. This determines a minor degree of immunological dysregulation with immunological reactivity to unidentified antigens, possibly microbial, such as cross-reacting antigens between the oral mucosa and *Streptococcus sanguis* or its L

form, or heat-shock protein. Cell-mediated immune mechanisms appear to be involved in the pathogenesis: helper T-cells predominate early on, with some natural killer cells. Cytotoxic cells then appear and there is evidence for an antibody-dependent cellular cytotoxicity reaction (Figure 32.1).

Etiological factors can include stress, trauma, various foods (nuts, chocolate, potato crisps) and cessation of tobacco smoking. A minority (about 10–20%) of patients attending outpatient clinics with RAS have an underlying hematinic deficiency, usually a low serum iron or ferritin, or deficiency of a B vitamin (e.g. folate or B12). Some women have RAS clearly related to the progestogen level fall in the luteal phase of the menstrual cycle, and regress in pregnancy.

Ulcers similar to aphthae (aphthous-like ulcers) are also seen in other conditions (Chapter 33).

Diagnostic features
History
Oral: Aphthae often begin with a tingling or burning sensation at the site of the future ulcer, progressing to form a red spot, followed by an ulcer.

Extraoral: None (by definition).

Clinical features
Oral: Aphthae typically:
- start in childhood or adolescence
- are multiple
- are ovoid or round
- recur
- have a yellowish depressed floor

- have a pronounced red inflammatory halo.

Aphthae may present different clinical appearances and behaviors.

Minor aphthae (Mikulicz's aphthae) (Figure 32.2) are:
- small, 2–4 mm in diameter
- last 7–10 days
- tend not to be seen on gingiva, palate or dorsum of tongue
- heal with no obvious scarring
- most patients develop not more than six ulcers at any single episode.

Major aphthae (Sutton's ulcers) are less common, much larger, and more persistent than minor aphthae, and can affect the soft palate and dorsum of tongue as well as other sites (Figure 32.3). Sometimes termed periadenitis mucosa necrotica recurrens (PMNR), major aphthae:
- can exceed 1 cm in diameter
- are most common on the palate, fauces and lips,
- can take months to heal
- may leave scars on healing
- at any one episode there are usually fewer than six ulcers present.

Herpetiform ulcers clinically resemble herpetic stomatitis (Figure 32.4). They:
- start as multiple pinpoint aphthae
- enlarge and fuse to produce irregular ulcers
- can be seen on any mucosa, but especially on the tongue ventrum.

Extraoral: The presence of extraoral manifestions means there is another diagnosis.

Differential diagnosis: From aphthous-like ulcers.

Investigations: There is no specific diagnostic test of value. Blood tests, to exclude identifiable causes, may include:
- full blood count
- hemoglobin assay
- white cell count and differential
- red cell indices
- iron studies
- red cell folate level
- serum vitamin B12 measurements
- serum anti-tissue transglutaminase antibodies.

Rarely, biopsy may be indicated to establish definitive diagnosis, since single aphthae may mimic carcinoma and pemphigus may start with aphthous-like ulceration. Histopathology shows an ulcer covered by fibrinous exudate infiltrated by polymorphonuclears overlying granulation tissue with dilated capillaries and edema over a fibroblastic repair reaction.

Management
Treatment aims are to:
- reduce pain
- reduce ulcer duration
- increase disease-free intervals.

Features that might suggest a systemic background, and indicate specialist referral (Figure 32.5) include:
- Any suggestion of systemic disease from extraoral features such as:
  — genital, skin or ocular lesions
  — gastrointestinal complaints (e.g. pain, altered bowel habits, blood in feces)
  — weight loss
  — weakness
  — chronic cough
  — fever
  — lymphadenopathy
  — hepatomegaly
  — splenomegaly
- An atypical history such as:
  — onset of ulcers in later adult life
  — exacerbation of ulceration
  — severe aphthae
  — aphthae unresponsive to topical hydrocortisone or triamcinolone
- Presence of other oral lesions, especially:
  — candidosis (including angular stomatitis)
  — glossitis
  — purpura or gingival bleeding
  — gingival swelling
  — necrotizing gingivitis
  — herpetic lesions
  — hairy leukoplakia
  — Kaposi sarcoma.

Predisposing factors should be corrected. If there is an obvious relationship to certain foods, the causal food should be excluded from the diet. Good oral hygiene should be maintained; chlorhexidine or triclosan mouthwashes help achieve this and may help reduce ulcer duration. Topical minocycline, doxycycline or other tetracycline mouth rinses may be of benefit.

Ulcer pain can usually be reduced, and the time to healing reduced, with hydrocortisone hemisuccinate pellets or triamcinolone acetonide in carboxymethylcellulose paste; failing the success of these, a stronger topical corticosteroid (e.g. beclometasone, betamethasone, clobetasol, fluticasone, mometasone) or systemic corticosteroid (e.g. prednisolone) may be required.

There are multiple other available therapies, including carbenoxolone, dapsone, cromoglicate, levamisole, colchicine, pentoxifylline, thalidomide and many others, but generally their efficacy has not been well proven or they have unacceptable adverse effects. Topical tacrolimus may be effective but randomized trials are awaited.

Prognosis
The natural history is of spontaneous resolution with age.

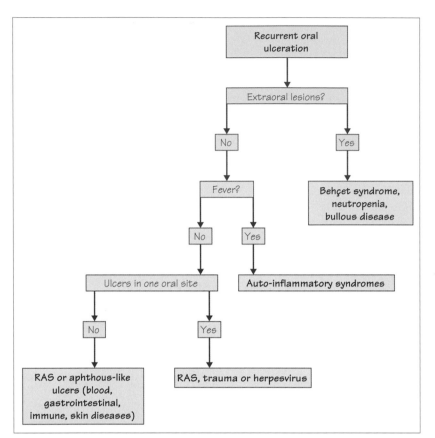

Figure 33.1 Recurrent ulcers diagnosis.

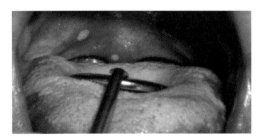

Figure 33.2 Behçet syndrome.

Table 33.1 Behçet syndrome manifestations.

Major	Minor
Mouth ulcers: (90–100% of cases)	Arthralgia
Genital ulcers	Thrombophlebitis – superficial or deep migratory
Ocular lesions	Intestinal lesions ; discrete bowel ulcerations
CNS lesions	Lung involvement; pneumonitis
Skin lesions and pathergy	Hematuria and proteinuria

Aphthous-like ulcers (ALU) are lesions that clinically resemble recurrent aphthous stomatitis but present atypically (e.g. commencement after adolescence, with fever, strong family history, or failing to resolve with age, or associated with systemic disease) (Figure 33.1).

Such ulcers may be seen in Behçet syndrome; immunodeficiencies, e.g. HIV/AIDS and neutropenias; autoinflammatory syndromes, e.g. periodic fever, aphthous stomatitis, pharyngitis and cervical adenitis (PFAPA); hematological diseases; gastrointestinal disorders; dermatological disorders; drugs; and infections such as HIV and infectious mononucleosis.

Behçet syndrome is especially important since the mouth ulcers so closely resemble aphthae, that it must be excluded in people who have recurrent mouth ulcers.

Behçet syndrome (BS, Behçet disease)

Definition: Aphthous-like ulcers associated with systemic disease.

Prevalence (approximate): Rare, most common in people from the Mediterranean and Middle East, Central Asia, China, Korea and Japan (the "silk road" from Europe to the Far East).

Age mainly affected: Young adults.

Gender mainly affected: M > F.

Etiopathogenesis: BS is an immunological disorder with a genetic background. There are familial cases and often associations with HLA-B5101. The many immunological findings include:
- T-helper (CD4) to T-suppressor (CD8) cell ratio decreased.
- Circulating autoantibodies against intermediate filaments, cardiolipin and neutrophil cytoplasm.
- Mononuclear cells initiate antibody-dependent cellular cytotoxicity to oral epithelial cells, and there is disturbed natural killer cell activity. Also involved are hyperactive polymorphonuclear leukocytes and cytokines (interleukins, tumor necrosis factor).
- Immune (antigen-antibody) complexes circulate and are deposited in blood vessel walls, initiating leukocytoclastic vasculitis. Many of the clinical features (erythema nodosum, arthralgia, uveitis) are common to established immune complex disease. The antigen responsible may include herpes simplex virus or streptococcal antigens. Heat-shock proteins have also been implicated.

Nearly all of the features of BS are due to the blood vessel inflammation which can produce widespread effects in many tissues, from mucosae, skin, and eyes (uvea and retina), to brain, blood vessels, joints, skin, and bowels.

Clinical features

Most patients present with oral, genital and ocular disease but many other tissues can be affected.

History

Oral: Recurrent ulcers.

Extraoral: Non-specific signs and symptoms may precede mucosal ulceration by up to five years. Sore throats, myalgias and migratory erythralgias are common. Malaise, anorexia, weight loss, weakness, headache, sweating, lymphadenopathy, large joint arthralgia and pain in substernal and temporal regions may occur.

Clinical features

Oral: Aphthous-like ulcers often affect the palate (Figure 33.2).

Extraoral: Genital, ocular, cutaneous, neurological, and vascular lesions are common.

Genitals: Ulcers resemble aphthae, affect the scrotum and penis of males and vulva of women and can scar.

Eyes: Impaired visual acuity; uveitis (anterior uveitis) with conjunctivitis (early) and hypopyon (late), retinal vasculitis (posterior uveitis), and optic atrophy. Both eyes are eventually involved and blindness may result.

Skin: Acneiform rashes; pustules at venepuncture sites (pathergy); pseudofolliculitis and erythema nodosum (tender red nodules over shins).

Neurological: Headache, psychiatric, motor or sensory manifestations; meningoencephalitis, cerebral infarction (stroke), psychosis, cranial nerve palsies, cerebellar and spinal cord lesions.

Venous thrombosis: Raised von Willebrand factor can cause thrombosis of large veins (vena cavae or dural sinuses).

Arthritis: Joint swelling, stiffness, pain, and tenderness occur in about half of patients at sometime during their lives. Most commonly affected are knees, wrists, ankles, and elbows.

Differential diagnosis: Inflammatory bowel diseases, connective tissue diseases, syphilis, Reiter syndrome (reactive arthritis).

Diagnosis

The diagnosis is difficult because:
- symptoms rarely appear simultaneously
- many other disorders have similar symptoms
- there is no single pathological diagnostic test to diagnose BS.

BS is therefore diagnosed clinically and there are three levels of certainty for diagnosis:

(1) International Study Group diagnostic guidelines (for research)
(2) Practical clinical diagnosis (generally agreed pattern)
(3) "Suspected" or "Possible" diagnosis (incomplete pattern of symptoms).

Practical clinical diagnostic criteria include recurrent oral ulceration (at least three episodes in 12 months) plus two or more other major manifestations (criteria: Table 33.1).

Findings of HLA-B5101 and pathergy are supportive of the diagnosis, as are antibodies to cardiolipin and neutrophil cytoplasm. Brain MRI may show focal lesions or enlargement of ventricles or subarachnoid spaces but can be normal even in the presence of neurological involvement. Biopsy of the skin or oral and genital ulcers is rarely indicated but reveals lymphocytic and plasma cell invasion in the prickle cell layer of the epithelium. Vessel walls show IgM and C3 immune deposits and, occasionally, necrotizing vasculitis.

Disease activity may be assessed by raised erythrocyte sedimentation rate, serum levels of acute phase proteins (e.g. CRP) or antibodies to intermediate filaments.

Management

BS rarely spontaneously remits. Patients with suspected BS should be referred early for specialist advice and treatment. Multidisciplinary care is often required, involving oral physicians, dermatologists, rheumatologists, ophthalmologists, neurologists, gynecologists and urologists.

Oral ulcers: Are treated as for aphthae.

Systemic manifestations: These are treated with aspirin, anticoagulants and immunosuppression (using colchicine, corticosteroids, azathioprine, ciclosporin, dapsone, rebamipide or pentoxifylline). Interferon alfa or anti-TNF therapy (e.g. thalidomide, infliximab, etanercept) are increasingly used.

Prognosis

BS has considerable morbidity especially in terms of ocular and neurological disease, with a relapsing and remitting but variable course. Mortality can occur from neurological, vascular, bowel, or cardiopulmonary involvement or as a complication of therapy.

Ulcers and erosions: Blood diseases, gastrointestinal disorders

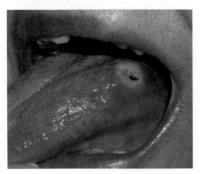

Figure 34.1 Leukemia.

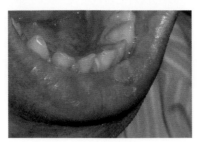

Figure 34.2 Aphthous-like ulcers in celiac disease.

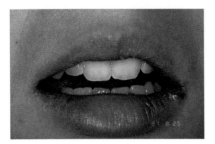

Figure 34.3 Unilateral angular stomatitis.

Table 34.1 Leukemias.

	Lymphocytic leukemia ("lymphoblastic")		Myelogenous leukemia ("myeloid" or "non-lymphocytic")	
Type	Acute lymphoblastic	Chronic lymphocytic	Acute myelogenous	Chronic myelogenous
Acronym	ALL	CLL	AML	CML
Age mainly affected	Most common childhood leukemia	Adults > 55	Adult males	Adults
Treatment	Chemotherapy and radiation	Chemotherapy and corticosteroids	Chemotherapy	Imatinib
% 5-year survival	85 in children 50 in adults	75	40	90

Aphthous-like and other mouth ulcers may be seen in disorders affecting the blood or gastrointestinal system.

Blood diseases

Ulcers may be seen in anemia and leukocyte defects (neutropenia, agranulocytopenia, leukemia, myelodysplastic syndromes or chronic granulomatous disease). In leukocyte defects there may also be severe gingivitis, rapid periodontal breakdown, as well as infections – mainly viral and fungal – and lymphadenopathy. Chemotherapy treatment and hematopoietic stem cell (bone marrow) transplantation can also produce oral ulceration and infections.

Leukemias

Definition: Malignant leukocyte proliferation (Greek leukos, "white"; aima, "blood"); there are several types (Table 34.1).

Prevalence (approximate): Uncommon.

Age mainly affected: 50–60% of leukemias are acute, affect mainly children or young adults. CML is seen mainly in middle-aged adults; CLL is seen mainly in the elderly.

Gender mainly affected: M = F.

Etiopathogenesis: Ionizing radiation, immunosuppression, chemicals (e.g. hair dyes; benzene), chromosomal disorders (e.g. Down syndrome), retroviruses (rarely). Fanconi anemia predisposes to AML.

Diagnostic features

History

Oral: Ulcers, infections.

Extraoral: Pallor, fatigue, bruising, infections.

Clinical features

Oral: Oral purpura (petechiae and ecchymoses) and spontaneous gingival hemorrhage.

Mouth ulcers: Associated with cytotoxic therapy, with viral, bacterial or fungal infection, or non-specific (Figure 34.1). Herpes simplex or zoster-varicella virus ulcers are common.

Microbial infections, mainly fungal and viral, are common in the mouth and can be a significant problem. Candidosis is extremely common. Herpes labialis is also common.

Simple odontogenic infections can spread widely and be difficult to control.

Non-odontogenic oral infections can involve a range of bacteria, including *Staphylococcus aureus*, *Pseudomonas aeruginosa*, *Klebsiella pneumoniae*, *Staphylococcus epidermidis*, *Escherichia coli*, and *Enterococcus* spp. especially in acute leukemias, and may act as a portal for septicemia.

Other occasional findings include mucosal pallor, paresthesia (particularly of the lower lip), facial palsy, extrusion of teeth or bone, painful swellings over the mandible and parotid swelling (Mikulicz syndrome). Leukemic deposits occasionally cause swelling, e.g. gingival swelling is a feature especially of myelomonocytic leukemia.

Extraoral: Anemia, purpura, infections, lymphadenopathy, hepatosplenomegaly.

Differential diagnosis: Other causes of ulcers and purpura.

Blood picture and bone marrow biopsy are mandatory investigations.

Management

Therapy for leukemia includes chemotherapy (Table 34.1), cladribine, pentostatin, rituximab, radiotherapy, bone marrow or stem cell transplant, monoclonal antibodies and corticosteroids. Supportive care includes oral hygiene and topical analgesics; aciclovir for herpetic infections; antifungals for candidosis.

Prognosis

Good for many, with a five-year survival rate about 50%. In children with ALL this is 85% (Table 34.1).

Gastrointestinal disorders

Malabsorption states (pernicious anemia, Crohn disease and celiac disease) may precipitate mouth ulcers in a small minority of patients. Oral lesions, termed pyostomatitis vegetans, are deep fissures, pustules and papillary projections seen rarely, mostly in patients with inflammatory bowel disease, i.e. ulcerative colitis or Crohn disease. The course of these lesions tends to follow that of the associated bowel disease. Although the oral lesions may respond partially to topical therapy (e.g. corticosteroids), systemic treatment is often needed.

Celiac disease (gluten sensitive enteropathy)

Definition: A hypersensitivity to gluten, affecting the small intestine (Greek, koiliakos = abdominal).

Prevalence (approximate): < 1% of the population, but more commonly in ethnic groups such as Celtic descendants, rare in people of African, Japanese and Chinese descent.

Age mainly affected: From childhood (not always recognized).

Gender mainly affected: M = F.

Etiopathogenesis: A genetically determined hypersensitivity to gliadin, a gluten protein constituent of wheat, barley and rye that affects the jejunum. Most patients have the variant HLA-DQ2 or DQ8 alleles (DQ2.5 has high frequency in peoples of North and Western Europe, where celiac disease is most common). Viral exposures, i.e. adenovirus type 12, may trigger an immunologic response in persons genetically susceptible to celiac disease.

Tissue transglutaminase modifies gliadin to a protein that causes an immunological cross-reaction with jejunal tissue, causing inflammation and loss of villi (villous atrophy), thus leading to malabsorption.

Diagnostic features

History

Oral: Ulcers, angular cheilitis or sore mouth. Symmetrically distributed enamel hypoplastic defects are common.

Extraoral: Patients may fail to thrive and/or have chronic diarrhea, or malabsorption (e.g. fatigue, anemia, osteopenia and sometimes a bleeding tendency) but many appear otherwise well. Associated autoimmune conditions such as diabetes mellitus type 1 and thyroid disease are common and dermatitis herpetiformis and/or IgA deficiency may occasionally be seen.

Clinical features

Oral: Perhaps 3% of patients with aphthous-like ulcers have celiac disease (Figure 34.2) and other oral features may include angular stomatitis (Figure 34.3); glossitis or burning mouth syndrome; and dental hypoplasia.

Extraoral: Symptomless or diarrhea and malabsorption, and weight loss.

Differential diagnosis: From inflammatory bowel disease.

A blood picture and hematinic assay results may suggest malabsorption, but the first-line investigation is assay of serum antibodies against tissue transaminase (anti-tTG), possibly followed by HLA-DQ2 and DQ8, and small bowel biopsy.

Management

Nutritional deficiencies should be rectified and the patient must thereafter adhere strictly to a gluten-free diet, i.e. no wheat, barley or rye, when oral lesions invariably resolve or ameliorate. Corn and rice are safe.

Prognosis

Good, but celiac disease predisposes to small intestine adenocarcinoma and lymphoma.

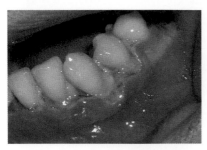

Figure 35.1 *Acute necrotizing gingivitis.*

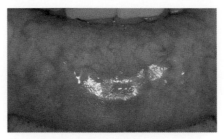

Figure 35.2 *Secondary syphilis.*

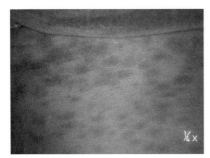

Figure 35.3 *Rash of secondary syphilis.*

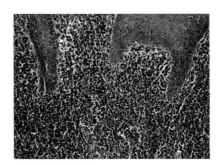

Figure 35.4 *Syphilis 20 ×.*

Herpesviruses and many other viruses can cause mouth ulceration (see Chapters 9 and 10) typically in children, and present with multiple ulcers and an acute febrile illness. EBV can also cause ulceration (see Chapter 60). Acute necrotizing gingivitis is a bacterial infection seen mainly where hygiene and/or nutrition are poor or in HIV/AIDS, especially in resource-poor areas. Chronic bacterial (e.g. syphilis, tuberculosis), fungal (e.g. histoplasmosis) and parasitic (e.g. leishmaniasis) infections may cause chronic ulceration, mainly in adults, again especially in resource-poor areas and in HIV/AIDS.

Hand, foot and mouth disease (HFM; vesicular stomatitis with exanthem)

Definition: Oropharyngeal vesicles and ulcers, with vesicles on hands and/or feet.

Prevalence (approximate): Uncommonly reported.

Age mainly affected: Children; epidemics common in Asia and Australia. Sometimes seen in immunocompromised adults.

Gender mainly affected: M = F.

Etiopathogenesis: Picornaviridae (Coxsackie virus A16 usually, but A5, A7, A9 and A10 or B9, or other enteroviruses).

Diagnostic features

History

Oral: Infection may be subclinical. The incubation period is up to a week. One or two days after fever onset, painful mouth sores develop.

Extraoral: Fever, headache, malaise, anorexia, diarrhea.

Clinical features

Oral: Shallow, painful, small ulcers mainly on tongue or buccal mucosa.

Extraoral: Non-itchy rash develops over 1–2 days on the palms of the hands and soles of the feet, sometimes also on buttocks and/or genitalia. The rash is of flat or raised red spots, sometimes with small, painful vesicles.

Differential diagnosis: Herpetic stomatitis; herpangina.

Investigations

This is a clinical diagnosis. Serology is confirmatory but rarely required.

Management

No specific treatment is available. Mouth lesions can be treated symptomatically. Skin vesicles heal spontaneously in about one week. Aspirin should be avoided in children.

Prognosis

Good. Small mortality from encephalitis, meningitis, paralysis, or pulmonary edema/hemorrhage.

Herpangina

Definition: An acute febrile illness associated with vesicles and ulcers in oropharynx (Latin, *herp* = an itch, *angina* = choking).

Prevalence (approximate): Uncommonly reported. Epidemics reported worldwide (most recently in Japan, with some fatalities).

Age mainly affected: Children.

Gender mainly affected: M = F.

Etiopathogenesis: Enteroviruses, mainly Coxsackie A1-A6, A8, A10, A12, A16 or A22, but similar syndromes can be caused by B1–5 and ECHOviruses (9 or 17).

Diagnostic features
History

Oral: Sore mouth.

Extraoral: Fever, malaise, headache, sore throat lasting 3–6 days.

Clinical features
Oral: Vesicular eruption mainly on fauces and soft palate, which rupture to leave round, painful, shallow ulcers.

Extraoral: None.

Differential diagnosis: Herpetic stomatitis; HFM.

Investigations
This is a clinical diagnosis. Coxsackievirus A may be recovered from the nasopharynx, feces, blood, urine, and cerebrospinal fluid.

Management
As for HFM.

Prognosis
Good. Rarely complicated by CNS lesions and cardiopulmonary failure.

Bacterial infections
Acute necrotizing ulcerative gingivitis (Vincent disease; acute ulcerative gingivitis, AUG, ANG, ANUG)

Definition: Painful gingival ulceration, affecting mainly the interdental papillae.

Prevalence (approximate): Uncommon, except in children in developing countries, especially Sub-Saharan Africa and India; 4–16% in HIV infected patients.

Age mainly affected: Young adults.

Gender mainly affected: M > F.

Etiopathogenesis: Proliferation of anaerobic fusiform bacteria and spirochaetes (variously *Borrelia vincentii*, *Fusobacterium necrophorum*, *Prevotella intermedia*, *Fusobacterum nucleatum*, *Porphyromonas gingivalis* as well as *Treponema* and *Selemonas* spp. and sometimes others. e.g. *Stenotrophomonas maltophilia*, *Pseudomonas aeruginosa*, *Bacteroides fragilis*, and *Staphylococcus aureus*). Predisposing factors include:
- poor oral hygiene
- smoking
- malnutrition
- immune defects.

Diagnostic features
History

Oral: Sore gingivae; bleeding, mouth odor.

Extraoral: None.

Clinical features
Oral: Painful ulceration starting on interdental papillae (Figure 35.1); pronounced gingival bleeding; halitosis; sialorrhea.

Extraoral: Occasional fever and cervical lymphadenopathy.

Differential diagnosis: Herpetic stomatitis, leukemia.

Investigations: Smear is optional.

Management
Oral debridement and hygiene instruction; peroxide or perborate mouthwashes; metronidazole (penicillin in pregnant females); periodontal assessment.

Prognosis
Good, but a rapid progression of the lesion to the cheek in malnourished or immunosuppressed patients with infection may lead to cancrum oris (noma, or "neglected third world disease").

Syphilis

In primary syphilis, a primary chancre (hard or Hunterian chancre) may involve the lip, tongue or palate. A small, firm, pink macule changes to a papule which ulcerates to form a painless round ulcer with a raised margin and indurated base. Chancres heal spontaneously in 3–8 weeks but are highly infectious and are associated with enlarged, painless regional lymph nodes.

In secondary syphilis, which follows after 6–8 weeks, about one-third of patients have highly infectious painless ulcers (mucous patches and snail-track ulcers) (Figure 35.2). Rash (Figure 35.3) and lymphadenopathy are common and lesions show a dense plasma cell infiltrate (Figure 35.4).

In tertiary syphilis a localized granuloma (gumma) that varies in size from a pinhead to several centimeters may arise, affecting particularly palate or tongue. Gummas break down to form deep chronic punched-out ulcers that are not infectious.

More common is leukoplakia on the dorsum of the tongue which has been considered as having a high potential for malignant change but this is contraversial.

Congenital syphilis may present with dental anomalies such as Hutchinson teeth.

Gonorrhea

Oropharyngeal asymptomatic carriage of gonococci is found in around 4% of those attending clinics for sexually transmitted infections. Mucosal erythema, sometimes with edema and ulceration may occur.

Tuberculosis

The most common oral presentation in pulmonary tuberculosis is a lump or chronic ulcer, usually of the dorsum of tongue, but jaw lesions or cervical lymphadenitis may be seen. Atypical mycobacterial ulcers, are caused particularly by *Mycobacterium avium-intracellulare*, often as a complication of HIV/AIDS, occasionally in apparently healthy individuals. Cervicofacial infection is occasionally caused by *M. chelonei*, usually as lymph node abscesses, or occasionally as intraoral swellings. Tuberculosis is a notifiable disease in the UK (the Proper Officer of the local authority must be notified).

36 Ulcers and erosions: Erythema multiforme, toxic epidermal necrolysis and Stevens-Johnson syndrome

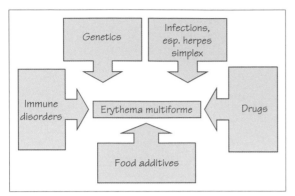

Figure 36.1 Erythema multiforme etiology.

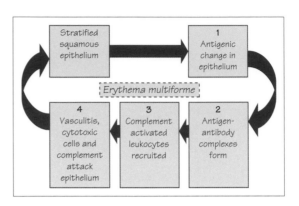

Figure 36.2 Erythema multiforme pathogenesis.

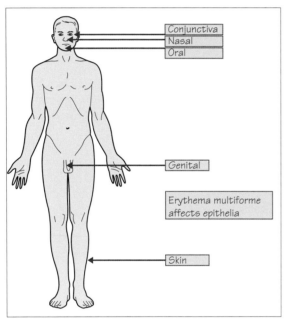

Figure 36.3 Erythema multiforme.

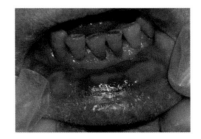

Figure 36.4 Erythema multiforme.

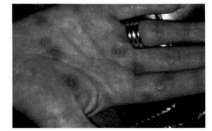

Figure 36.5 Erythema multiforme target lesions.

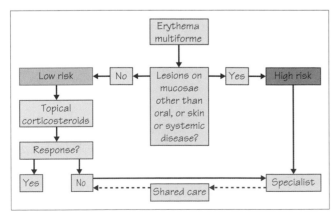

Figure 36.6 Erythema multiforme treatment.

Table 36.1 Main causal factors in erythema multiforme.

Micro-organisms	Drugs*	Chemicals	Immune factors
Herpes simplex virus	Allopurinol	Benzoates	BCG
Mycoplasma pneumoniae	Aminopenicillins	Nitrobenzene	Graft versus host diseases
	Anticonvulsants	Perfumes	Hepatitis B immunization
	Barbiturates	Terpenes	Inflammatory bowel disease
	Cephalosporins		Polyarteritis nodosa
	Corticosteroids		Sarcoidosis
	Quinolones		Systemic lupus erythematosus
	Oxicam NSAIDS		
	Protease inhibitors		
	Sulfonamides		

* Incriminated in TEN (toxic epidermal necrolysis) and SJS (Stevens-Johnson syndrome).

Erythema multiforme

Definition: Erythema multiforme (EM) is a mucocutaneous condition mediated by antigen-antibody (immune complex – mainly IgM) deposition in the superficial microvasculature of skin and mucous membranes.

Prevalence (approximate): Uncommon.

Age mainly affected: Younger adults in second and third decades.

Gender mainly affected: M > F.

Etiopathogenesis: There may be a genetic predisposition, with various HLA associations (e.g. patients with extensive mucosal involvement may have HLA-DQB1*0402). A putative immunological hypersensitivity reaction usually to various micro-organisms or drugs (Figure 36.1) (Table 36.1), results in immune complexes and the ingress of cytotoxic CD8 T lymphocytes, inducing keratinocyte apoptosis and satellite cell necrosis (Figure 36.2).

Diagnostic features

EM minor (accounts for 80%) is a mild, self-limiting rash usually affecting one mucosa. EM major is a severe, life-threatening variant that overlaps with toxic epidermal necrolysis (see below) and involves multiple mucous membranes and epithelia (Figure 36.3).

History

Oral: Often recurrent attacks, classically with serosanguinous exudates on the lips for 10–14 days once or twice a year.

Extraoral: EM minor may cause a mild rash. EM major causes widespread lesions also affecting eyes, pharynx, larynx, esophagus, skin and genitals, with bullous, target-like lesions and other rashes, pneumonia, arthritis, nephritis or myocarditis.

Clinical features

Oral: Most patients with EM (70%), of either minor or major forms, have oral lesions which begin as erythematous macules that blister and break down to irregular, extensive, painful erosions with extensive surrounding erythema, typically most pronounced in the anterior mouth (Figure 36.4). The labial mucosa is often involved, and a serosanguinous exudate leads to crusting of the swollen lips.

Extraoral: Rash; typically target, or iris-like (Figure 36.5) but, in EM major, may be bullous.

Ocular changes: Resemble those of pemphigoid; dry eyes and symblepharon may result.

Genital changes: Include balanitis, urethritis and vulval ulcers.

Differential diagnosis: Viral stomatitides, pemphigus, toxic epidermal necrolysis and subepithelial immune blistering disorders (pemphigoid and others).

Investigations: The diagnosis is mainly clinical; the Nikolsky sign is negative. There are no specific diagnostic tests. HLA-DQ3 may be a helpful marker for distinguishing herpes-associated EM from other diseases with EM-like lesions. Blood tests may be helpful (serology for *Mycoplasma pneumoniae* or HSV (or DNA or immunostain studies), or other micro-organisms).

Biopsy/histopathology of perilesional tissue with immunostaining and histological examination may help but not invariably, since the histopathology is extremely variable. The most typical features are intraepithelial blisters due to areas of intercellular edema, which coalesce to form vesicles. There is a variable inflammatory reaction in the corium, sometimes with subepithelial vesiculation. Thus there may be intra- or subepithelial vesiculation. Sometimes eosinophilic coagula develop within the upper epithelium, forming large, round, eosinophilic bodies which are fibrinous in nature. True vasculitis is rare in early lesions but sometimes there is a perivascular infiltrate. In later lesions there is perivascular cuffing and sometimes vasculitis, and the whole epithelium becomes necrotic and sloughs. When there is an extensive inflammatory overlay the interpretation is difficult. Immunostaining shows fibrin and C3 at the epithelial basement membrane zone, and perivascular IgM, C3 and fibrin, but is not specific.

Management

Spontaneous healing can be slow, taking up to 2–3 weeks in EM minor and up to six weeks in EM major, and thus treatment is indicated and specialist care may be required (Figure 36.6). No specific therapy is available but supportive care is important; a liquid diet and even intravenous fluid therapy may be necessary. Oral hygiene should be improved with 0.2% aqueous chlorhexidine mouthbaths. The use of corticosteroids is controversial:

• EM minor may respond to topical corticosteroids, although systemic corticosteroids may still be required.

• EM major should be treated with systemic corticosteroids (prednisolone) and/or azathioprine, ciclosporin, levamisole, thalidomide or other immunomodulatory drugs.

Antimicrobials may be indicated.

• Aciclovir or valaciclovir is used in herpes-associated EM.

• Tetracycline is used in EM related to *Mycoplasma pneumoniae*.

Prognosis

Most cases resolve without sequelae in 2–4 weeks. Some recur.

Toxic epidermal necrolysis (TEN, Lyell syndrome) and Stevens-Johnson syndrome (SJS)

Toxic epidermal necrolysis (TEN) is a rare, potentially lethal mucocutaneous condition in which the skin peels off in swaths, with 30% or more epithelial detachment. Stevens-Johnson syndrome (SJS) is a milder form, with epithelial detachment involving less than 10% of body surface. Both TEN and SJS usually affect the mouth, and early on. They involve two or more mucosal surfaces and present with blisters that arise on erythematous or purpuric macules. Fever is common. Mucous membrane involvement can result in gastrointestinal hemorrhage, respiratory failure, and ocular and genitourinary complications.

Typically these conditions arise as adverse drug reactions (e.g. to NSAIDs, allopurinol, antiretrovirals, anticonvulsants (including carbamazepine) or sulfonamides). Most cases occur within the first four weeks of drug exposure. Family members may also react similarly if exposed to the offending drug. There is a strong association between HLA-B*1502 and carbamazepine-induced TEN among Han Chinese. These conditions must be differentiated mainly from paraneoplastic syndromes, and the staphylococcal scalded skin syndrome.

Treatment is withdrawal of culprit drugs, and urgent specialist referral to a burns or intensive care unit for treatment (with intravenous immunoglobulins, ciclosporin, cyclophosphamide, plasmapheresis, infliximab, ulinastatin (protease inhibitor of neutrophil elastase) or pentoxyfylline), supportive management, and nutritional support.

Prognosis

TEN is fatal in 30% and SJS in 5% of cases.

37

White lesions: Candidosis (candidiasis)

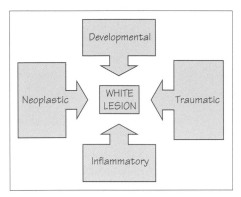

Figure 37.1 *Causes of white lesions.*

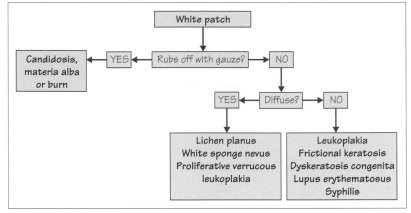

Figure 37.2 *White patch diagnosis.*

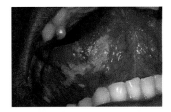

Figure 37.3 *Factors predisposing to candidosis.*

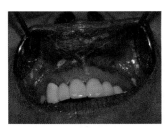

Figure 37.4 *Pseudomembranous candidosis.*

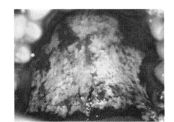

Figure 37.5 *Candidosis.*

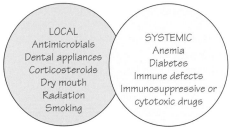

Figure 37.6a *Candidosis in HIV/AIDS before wiping with gauze.*

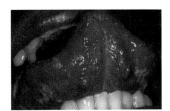

Figure 37.6b *Candidosis after wiping with gauze.*

Table 37.1 *Causes of oral white lesions.*

Acquired				
Infective	**Mucocutaneous diseases**	**Neoplastic and possibly pre-neoplastic**	**Others**	**Developmental**
Candidosis and candidal leukoplakia Hairy leukoplakia Koplik spots (early measles) Papillomas Syphilitic leukoplakia	Lichen planus and lichenoid lesions Lupus erythematosus	Carcinoma Leukoplakias	Burns Friction Grafts Materia alba	Darier disease Dyskeratosis congenita Pachyonychia congenita White sponge nevus

White patches may be produced by epithelial debris (e.g. "material alba" – white debris which accumulates where oral hygiene is lacking), sloughing (e.g. burns), or epithelial thickening – rarely inherited but more commonly acquired (Figure 37.1) (Table 37.1). Superficial conditions such as debris or candidosis can be wiped away with a dry gauze (Figure 37.2).

Acute pseudomembranous candidosis

(Also called "thrush" in UK and some other countries.)

Definition: Lesions consist of white flecks, plaques or nodules, which will wipe off with gauze.

Prevalence (approximate): Uncommon.

Age mainly affected: Neonates and adults.

Gender mainly affected: M = F.

Etiopathogenesis: *Candida albicans* is a harmless commensal yeast in the mouths of nearly 50% of the population (carriers). Oropharyngeal candidosis may be seen in healthy neonates as they have yet to acquire immunity. Local ecological changes such as a disturbance in the oral flora (e.g. by antibiotics, xerostomia), or a decrease in immune defences (e.g. by immunosuppressive treatment or immune defects (HIV/AIDS, leukemias, lymphomas, cancer, diabetes)), can allow *Candida* to become an *opportunistic* pathogen (Figure 37.3). There is also an increase in non-albicans species (e.g. *Candida glabrata*, *C. tropicalis*, *C. krusei*).

Diagnostic features

History

Oral: Sometimes soreness.

Extraoral: Soreness.

Clinical features

Oral: Candidosis presents anywhere but especially in the upper buccal vestibule (Figure 37.4) and the palate (Figure 37.5). White or creamy plaques that can be wiped off to leave a red base are typical (Figures 37.6a and b). Red lesions may occur. Lesions may thus be white, mixed white and red, or red.

Extraoral: Other mucosae, nails and skin may be affected if the cause is generalized, such as an immune defect.

Differential diagnosis: Lichen planus, hairy leukoplakia, leukoplakia, Koplik or Fordyce spots.

Investigations

The diagnosis is clinical usually, but a Periodic acid Schiff (PAS) or Gram-stained smear (hyphae) or oral rinse may help. Visible hyphae or blastospheres on potassium hydroxide mount indicate *Candida* infection. Culture is diagnostic.

Blood tests for an immune defect may be warranted.

Management

Treat predisposing cause and, for mild to moderate cases in otherwise healthy people, give two weeks of topical antifungals such as nystatin oral suspension or ointment (for perioral), or amphotericin lozenges, or miconazole oral gel or mucoadhesive buccal tablets. In moderate to severe cases, or the immunocompromised, fluconazole, itraconazole or voriconazole are indicated. In refractory cases, check to ensure that the patient is not immunocompromised or the organism is not azole-resistant.

Prognosis

Depends on cause.

Chronic hyperplastic candidosis (Candidal leukoplakia)

Definition: Leukoplakia and/or erythroplakia associated with candidosis.

Prevalence (approximate): Uncommon.

Age mainly affected; Middle-age and older.

Gender mainly affected: M = F.

Etiopathogenesis: *Candida albicans* can produce nitrosamines and can induce epithelial proliferation and dysplasia. Co-factors, such as smoking, vitamin deficiency and immune suppression, may contribute.

Diagnostic features

History

Oral: Often symptomless.

Clinical features

Oral: A tough adherent white leukoplakia-like plaque. The plaque is variable in thickness and often rough or irregular in texture, or nodular with an erythematous background (speckled leukoplakia). The usual sites are the dorsum of the tongue or the post-commissural buccal mucosa.

Differential diagnosis: Thrush, leukoplakia, keratosis, lichen planus.

Investigations

The plaque cannot be wiped off, but fragments can be detached by firm scraping. PAS or Gram-staining then show candidal hyphae embedded in clumps of detached epithelial cells. Biopsy/histopathology are indicated, and show a parakeratotic plaque infiltrated by polymorphs, spongiform pustules, and acanthosis. The candidal hyphae may not be easily seen in the hematoxylin and eosin stained slide but as in acute candidosis are readily visualized with PAS. The epithelium shows downgrowths of blunt or club-shaped rete ridges and there is thinning of the suprapapillary epithelium with a resemblance to psoriasis ("psoriasiform hyperplasia"). The basement membrane zone may be thick and prominent and there is variable inflammation in the corium.

Management and prognosis

Candidal leukoplakia may be potentially malignant. Persons with leukoplakia should be advised to stop any tobacco/alcohol/betel habits, and should be encouraged to have a diet rich in fruit and vegetables.

Antifungal treatment is indicated but, if the lesion fails to resolve, it is best to remove it by excision or laser.

Chronic mucocutaneous candidosis (CMC)

Definition: A heterogeneous group of syndromes characterized by persistent cutaneous, oral and other mucosal candidosis, with little propensity for systemic dissemination.

Prevalence (approximate): Rare.

Age mainly affected: From early pre-school childhood.

Gender mainly affected: M = F.

Etiopathogenesis: Various, usually congenital, cellular immune defects underly CMC, sometimes generalized, sometimes restricted to *Candida* (this is not one single entity). Decreased interleukin 2 (IL-2) and interferon-gamma (T_H 1 cytokines) and increased IL-10 may be implicated.

Hypoparathyroidism (with dental defects), diabetes, hypoadrenocorticism, and hypothyroidism may be seen in one variant – candidosis-endocrinopathy syndrome (CES). Autoimmune polyendocrinopathy-candidosis-ectodermal dystrophy (APECED) has significant morbidity from endocrinopathies or other autoimmune diseases. In thymoma (thymus tumor) and diseases such as myasthenia gravis, myositis, aplastic anemia, neutropenia and hypogammaglobulinemia, CMC may develop in adult life.

Diagnostic features

History

Oral: Symptomless or sore.

Extraoral: Symptomless or sore.

Clinical features

Oral: White plaques which become widespread, thick and adherent. Oral carcinoma may occasionally supervene.

Extraoral: Candidal infections of nails (paronychia and onychomycosis), scalp, trunk, hands and feet. HPV infections may also be prevalent.

Differential diagnosis: Candidosis, lichen planus, leukoplakia.

Investigations: Immunological testing, endocrinological testing.

Management

Sytemic antifungals.

Prognosis

Lesions tend to recur and *Candida* readily becomes drug-resistant but disseminated invasive infections and mycotic aneurysms are rare.

38

White lesions: Keratosis, leukoplakia

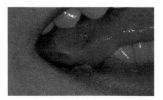

Figure 38.1 Biting causing keratosis.

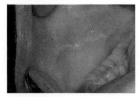

Figure 38.2 Biting mucosa causing keratosis.

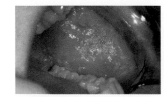

Figure 38.3 Cheek chewing.

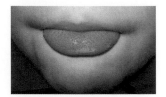

Figure 38.4 Frictional keratosis.

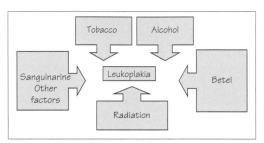

Figure 38.5 Leukoplakia etiology.

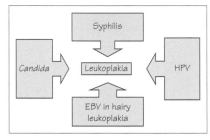

Figure 38.6 Leukoplakia: infective causes.

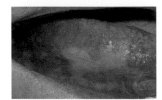

Figure 38.7 Homogeneous leukoplakia.

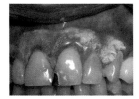

Figure 38.8 Verrucous leukoplakia.

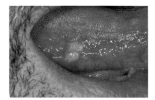

Figure 38.9 Leukoplakia that proved to be carcinoma.

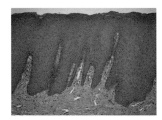

Figure 38.10a Acanthosis and hyperparakeratosis.

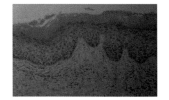

Figure 38.10b Keratosis and atrophy.

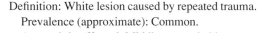

Figure 38.11 Leukoplakia management.

Definition: White lesion caused by repeated trauma.

Prevalence (approximate): Common.

Age mainly affected: Middle-age and older.

Gender mainly affected: M > F.

Etiopathogenesis: Etiological factors include prolonged abrasion (e.g. sharp tooth, dental appliance, toothbrushing, mastication, cheek biting). Bilateral alveolar ridge keratosis (BARK) may be seen in edentulous areas. An occlusal line (linea alba) is often seen on the lateral tongue (Figure 38.1) and in the buccal mucosae (Figure 38.2), as is cheek-biting (morsicatio buccarum or morsicatio mucosa oris, MMO), most prevalent in anxious females (Figure 38.3). Rarely self-mutilation is seen in psychiatric disorders (Figure 38.4), learning impairment or some rare syndromes.

Diagnostic features

Clinical features

Linea alba is typically thin, white with occasional petechiae and may be seen in isolation or sometimes with crenation of the margins of the tongue, from pressure. Cheek-biting causes white and red lesions with a shredded surface, in the labial and/or buccal mucosa near the occlusal line. Keratoses on edentulous ridges (BARK), especially in the partially dentate, are presumably caused by friction from mastication.

Differential diagnosis: Leukoplakia, lichen planus, leukoedema, white-sponge nevus, smokeless tobacco keratosis, chemical keratosis, and hairy leukoplakia.

The diagnosis is clinical. Histopathology can confirm lack of dysplasia and shows acanthosis and hyperkeratosis (usually orthokeratosis); spinous layer cells often demonstrate intraepithelial edema and occasional vacuolated cells resembling koilocytes.

Management

Apart from removing irritants and ceasing habits, no treatment is required.

Prognosis

There is no evidence that continued minor trauma alone has any carcinogenic potential.

Tobacco-related keratosis

Definition: White hyperkeratotic lesions caused by tobacco-chewing or snuff-dipping.

Prevalence (approximate): Uncommon.

Age mainly affected: Adults.

Gender mainly affected: M = F.

Etiopathogenesis: Tobacco-chewing or snuff-dipping (holding flavored tobacco powder in the vestibule) causes white edematous and hyperkeratotic wrinkled white plaque lesions (verrucous keratoses) in up to 20% of users. Oral snuff appears to cause more severe clinical changes than does tobacco-chewing, but dysplasia is more likely in chewers. Lesions can, after several decades of use, progress to verrucous carcinoma.

Diagnostic features

Clinical features

Oral: Typically a white lesion in the buccal sulcus adjacent to where snuff is placed, often with some gingival recession.

Differential diagnosis: Leukoplakia, lichen planus, leukoedema.

The diagnosis is usually obvious from the habit, but biopsy/histopathology may be reassuring in excluding dysplasia. Biopsy shows pronounced hyperparakeratosis and intraepithelial edema in the superficial epithelium.

Management

The patient should stop the habit.

Prognosis

Snuff dippers' lesions usually resolve on stopping the habit, even after 25 years of use, but any residual keratosis after two months should be considered a leukoplakia and viewed with suspicion.

Leukoplakia

Definition: "A predominantly white lesion of the oral mucosa that cannot be characterized as any other definable lesion" – a clinical term, without any histological connotation, to characterize white lesions that cannot be rubbed off with gauze or diagnosed as another specific disease entity. Leukoplakia is a potentially malignant disorder; it does not include frictional lesions or those associated with restorations or cheek-biting.

Prevalence (approximate): Up to 3% of adults.

Age mainly affected: Adults.

Gender mainly affected: M > F.

Etiopathogenesis: Most affected patients use tobacco or betel or drink alcohol (Figure 38.5). Less common identified causes include infections such as candidosis, syphilis and HPV (Figure 38.6). Dietary fibre, fruit and vegetables appear to be protective.

Where a specific etiological factor cannot be identified, the term *idiopathic* leukoplakia is used.

Diagnostic features

History

Oral: Most are symptomless.

Clinical features

Oral: May occur as white single localized, multiple, or diffuse widespread lesions. Most are smooth plaques (homogeneous leukoplakias) (Figure 38.7) seen on the lip, buccal mucosae, or gingivae; others are non-homogeneous. Of these some are warty (verrucous leukoplakia) (Figure 38.8); some are mixed white and red lesions (speckled leukoplakias or erythroleukoplakia). Whether homogeneous and non-homogeneous leukoplakias are independent disease entities or a continuum of progressive clinical phases is unclear.

A poorer prognosis is suggested by:
- surface nodularity
- erythema
- ulceration
- increased firmness and induration
- unexplained hemorrhage.

Differential diagnosis: Carcinoma, lichen planus, chronic cheek-biting, keratosis, stomatitis nicotina, leukoedema, white sponge nevus.

Investigations

Biopsy is mandatory; histological findings range from hyperkeratosis and hyperplasia to atrophy and dysplasia to carcinoma (Figure 38.9). Histopathological evidence of dysplasia is not a requirement for the diagnosis (Figures 38.10a and b), but appears to be the feature most predictive of malignant potential. The most appropriate area to biopsy is not easy; guidance can be obtained by selecting any associated *red* area or using toluidine blue staining (Chapter 3).

Management and prognosis

Persons with leukoplakia should be advised to stop any tobacco/alcohol/betel habits, and should be encouraged to have a diet rich in fruit and vegetables (70% of lesions then disappear or regress within 12 months).

The malignant transformation rates range from 3 to 33% over 15 years; up to 10% of those with moderate and 25% of those with severe dysplasia develop carcinoma in a ten-year period (estimated annual cancer rate 1%). Dysplasia appears to be the best predictor. Dysplastic lesions do not have any specific clinical appearance but, where erythroplasia is present, or the lesions are verrucous or nodular or speckled, then severe dysplasia or carcinomas may be seen. Site is also relevant; leukoplakias in the floor of mouth/ventrum of tongue and lip appear to be the most sinister. The most extensive follow-up studies suggest that idiopathic leukoplakia has the highest risk of developing cancer; malignant change appears to be more frequent among *non*-smokers.

Any dysplasia must be taken seriously but, even in studies of leukoplakias which on incisional biopsy showed *no* dysplasia but were excised, up to 10% had carcinoma in the excision specimens. Most experts therefore remove these lesions (with scalpel or laser) (Figure 38.11). Occasionally patients are treated by cryosurgery, photodynamic therapy or topical cytotoxic agents (e.g. bleomycin).

The patient should be followed regularly (at 6–12 months intervals).

39 White lesions: Hairy leukoplakia, lichen planus

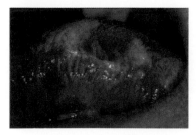

Figure 39.1 Hairy leukoplakia.

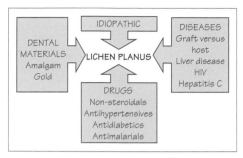

Figure 39.2 Lichen planus and lichenoid lesions etiology.

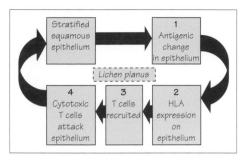

Figure 39.3 Lichen planus pathogenesis.

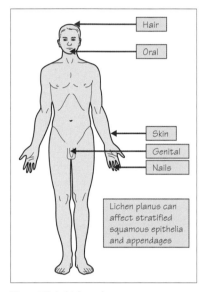

Figure 39.4 Lichen planus.

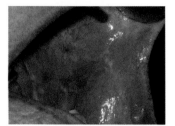

Figure 39.5a Lichen planus.

Figure 39.5b Lichen planus.

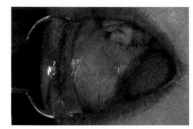

Figure 39.6 Lichen planus.

Figure 39.7 Lichen planus.

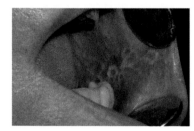

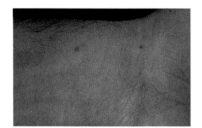

Figure 39.8 Histological features of LP.

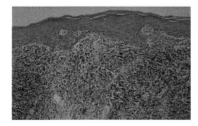

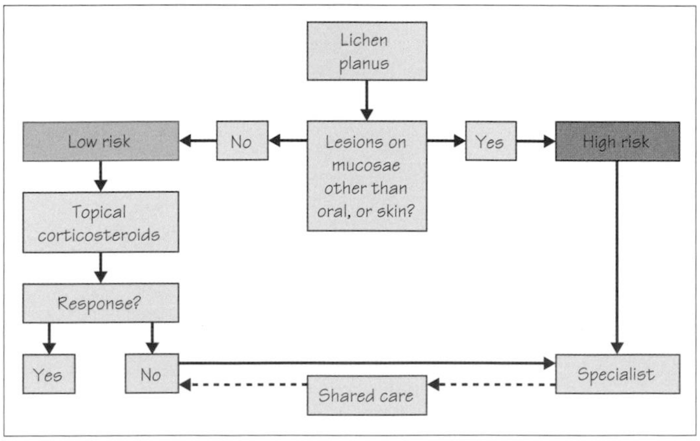

Figure 39.9 Lichen planus management.

Hairy leukoplakia

Definition: Bilateral white tongue lesions.

Prevalence (approximate): Uncommon.

Age mainly affected: Adult.

Gender mainly affected: M > F.

Etiopathogenesis: Epstein-Barr virus, usually in an immunocompromised patient, especially in HIV/AIDS. Cases have been reported in patients with hematological malignancies or organ transplants.

Diagnostic features

Clinical features

Oral: Vertically corrugated symptomless white lesions on the margins, dorsal or ventral surfaces of the tongue (Figure 39.1).

Extraoral: Maybe lesions of HIV/AIDS or immunodeficiency.

Differential diagnosis: Frictional keratosis, lichen planus, tobacco-associated leukoplakia, geographic tongue.

Investigations

- HIV serotest.
- Biopsy/histopathology shows irregular parakeratosis and vacuolated cells with dark pyknotic nuclei (koilocytes-like) in the stratum spinosum.

Epithelial nuclei stain positively immunocytochemically and *in situ* hybridization for EBV capsid antigen.

Management
Anti-retroviral (ART) and anti-herpes agents (mainly valaciclovir and famciclovir) may clear the lesion. Topical therapy with podophyllin 25% and retinoids may also help. Cryotherapy has been reported as successful.

Prognosis
Appears to be benign, and self-limiting, but recurrences are common.

Lichen planus (LP) and lichenoid reactions
Definition: A mucocutaneous disorder characterized variably by oral, genital and/or skin lesions.

Prevalence (approximate): Possibly 1% of the population.

Age mainly affected: Middle-age and older.

Gender mainly affected: F > M.

Etiopathogenesis: A minority of cases have an identifiable offending agent such as drugs (e.g. antihypertensives, antidiabetics, gold salts, non-steroidal anti-inflammatory agents, antimalarials) or dental materials (amalgam, gold or others), or may arise in graft-versus-host disease (GVHD), HIV infection or hepatitis C (Figure 39.2). These are often termed lichenoid lesions. The etiology in most patients, however, is unclear (idiopathic LP).

Upregulation of epithelial basement membrane extracellular matrix proteins and the secretion of cytokines and intercellular adhesion molecules by keratinocytes facilitates ingress of T-lymphocytes which attack stratified squamous epithelia (Figure 39.3). Auto-cytotoxic CD8+ T-cells bind to keratinocytes and trigger the programmed cell death (apoptosis) of basal cells via tumor-necrosis factor alpha (TNF-alpha) and interferon gamma (IFN-gamma). TNF-alpha stimulates activation of nuclear factor kappa B (NF-kB) and production of inflammatory cytokines.

Inhibition of transforming growth factor beta which normally causes keratinocyte proliferation can lead to atrophic forms of LP. Genetic polymorphism of IFN-gamma is a risk factor for development of oral lesions, whereas TNF-alpha allele may be a risk factor for LP affecting mouth and skin.

Diagnostic features
History
Oral: Lesions may be asymptomatic or may cause soreness, especially if atrophic or erosive.

Extraoral: Typically an itchy rash, or genital soreness (Figure 39.4).

Clinical features
Oral: Typically, lesions are:
• bilateral
• posterior in the buccal (cheek) mucosa
• sometimes on the tongue, floor of mouth or gingivae
• rare on the palate

Presentations typically include white:
• network of raised white lines or striae (reticular pattern) (Figures 39.5a–b and Figure 39.6)
• papules
• plaques, simulating leukoplakia

Erosions are less common, persistent, irregular, and painful, with a yellowish slough (plus white lesions). Red atrophic areas and/or desquamative gingivitis may be seen.

Some lesions may be associated with hyperpigmentation.

Lichenoid oral lesions clinically and histologically resemble LP but may:
• be unilateral
• be associated with erosions
• affect particularly the palate and tongue.

Extraoral: LP may also affect:
• Skin; itchy (pruritic), purple, polygonal, papules especially on the flexor surface of the wrists (Figure 39.7). These may have white Wickham striae. Trauma may induce lesions (Koebner phenomenon).
• Genitals; white or erosive lesions (if there is also oral involvement, these are termed vulvovaginal-gingival or penile-gingival syndromes).
• Esophagus; white or erosive lesions.
• Nails; ridging.
• Hair; loss.

Differential diagnosis: Lupus erythematosus, leukoplakia, keratosis, malignancy, chronic ulcerative stomatitis, pemphigus, pemphigoid.

Investigations
Optional Blood tests may help exclude liver disease (hepatitis C) and diabetes.

Biopsy/histopathology; history and clinical appearance are usually highly indicative of the diagnosis but lesional biopsy is often indicated, particularly to differentiate from other conditions and exclude malignancy. Histological features of LP may include (Figure 39.8):
• a dense subepithelial cellular infiltrate including mostly T-lymphocytes
• hyperkeratosis and thickening of the granular cell layer
• basal cell liquefaction degeneration and colloid bodies
• "saw-tooth" appearance of rete pegs
• immunostaining for fibrin at the epithelial basement membrane zone.

It can be a problem in histopathology to characterize lichen, lichenoid and microscopically similar lesions, including sometimes leukoplakia.

Management
Predisposing factors should be excluded. If amalgams might be implicated, it may be worthwhile considering removing them. If drugs are implicated, the physician should be consulted as to possible alternatives.

Oral lesions may respond to the more potent topical corticosteroids (e.g. clobetasol, beclomethasone, or budesonide). Antifungals may be helpful.

Widespread, or severe, or recalcitrant lesions can be managed with intralesional or stronger topical corticosteroids.

Specialist referral may be indicated if there is concern about malignancy, extraoral lesions, diagnosis, or recalcitrant oral lesions (Figure 39.9). Topical tacrolimus or ciclosporin, or systemic immuno-suppressive agents (e.g. corticosteroids, azathioprine, ciclosporin or dapsone) or vitamin A derivatives (e.g. isotretinoin) may be required.

Persons with lichen planus should be advised to stop any tobacco/alcohol/betel habits, and should be encouraged to have a diet rich in fruit and vegetables.

Prognosis
Oral LP is often persistent but benign. Although controversial it is generally accepted that there is about a < 3% chance of malignant transformation over five years, predominantly in those with long-standing LP.

40

Salivary conditions: Salivary swelling and salivary excess

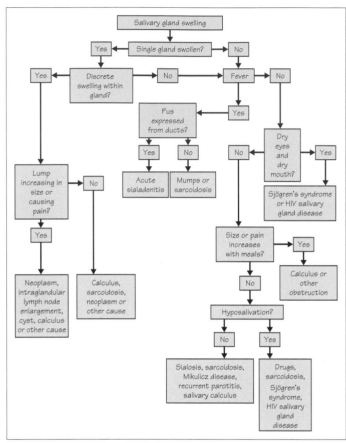

Figure 40.1 Diagnosis of salivary swelling.

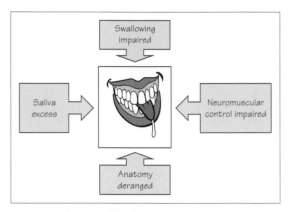

Figure 40.2 Causes of drooling.

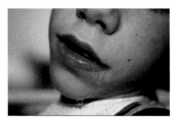

Figure 40.3 Drooling in learning impairment.

Box 40.1 Causes of excess saliva.

Psychogenic (usually)
Painful lesions in the mouth
Drugs or poisoning
Foreign bodies in the mouth
Poor neuromuscular coordination
Others

Table 40.1 Causes of salivary gland swelling.

Duct obstruction	Inflammatory	Neoplasms	Hypertrophy	Deposits	Drugs
Calculus (sialolithiasis)	Actinomycosis	Salivary	Sialosis (sialadenosis)	Amyloidosis	Antihypertensives
Mucus plug	Ascending sialadenitis	Other		Hemochromatosis	Chlorhexidine
Other	Lymphadenitis				Cytotoxic drugs
	Mikulicz disease (lymphoepithelial lesion and syndrome)				Iodine
	Radiation sialadenitis				
	Recurrent parotitis				
	Sarcoidosis				
	Sjögren syndrome				
	Tuberculosis				
	Viral sialadenitis				

Perhaps 700–1000 ml of saliva are produced each day, most by the parotid, submandibular and sublingual glands (major salivary glands).

Parotid saliva makes the bulk of the stimulated saliva and the submandibular gland produces 70% of resting saliva. Mucus glands (minor salivary glands) in the lips, palate and elsewhere produce mainly mucin and immunoglobulin A (IgA). Functions of saliva include facilitating lubrication in the mouth, pharynx and esophagus, and assisting swallowing, speech, digestion (amylase), and defense against infections (mainly IgA, lysozyme and histatins).

Saliva is produced in response to taste, masticatory or psychogenic stimuli. Control is mainly via the parasympathetic innervation.

The main complaints related to salivary glands are dry mouth and pain, but sialorrhea and salivary gland swelling (Table 40.1) can be concerns.

Salivary swelling

Swellings may be caused by salivary gland duct obstruction (e.g. stone/calculus); inflammation (e.g. sialadenitis; HIV/AIDS; Sjögren syndrome; sarcoidosis); neoplasm; sialosis; deposits; drugs; because of tumor infiltration from elsewhere, or because of salivary lymph node enlargement.

An algorithm for diagnosis of swellings is shown in Figure 40.1. The diagnosis of salivary complaints is from the history and examination often supplemented by investigations, especially imaging (Table 40.2). Fine needle aspiration (FNA) is useful to determine if a major gland enlargement is caused by tumor, lymphoma or reactive process. Labial gland biopsy may assist in diagnosis of Sjögren syndrome.

Saliva excess (sialorrhea, hypersialia, hypersalivation, ptyalism) and drooling

Sialorrhea describes increased salivary flow: *Drooling* is the overflowing of saliva from the mouth not usually associated with increased saliva production.

Causes: Painful lesions or foreign bodies in the mouth, drugs (e.g. anticholinesterases (insecticides and nerve agents); antipsychotics, and cholinergic agonists used to treat dementia and myasthenia gravis); toxins (e.g. mercury and thallium); and rarely other causes (e.g. rabies) may be implicated. Sialorrhea is an uncommon subjective complaint but objective evidence is even less common, and the problem is sometimes perceived rather than real. Causes of sialorrhea are shown in Box 40.1.

Drooling is normal in healthy infants, but usually stops by about 18 months and is considered abnormal if it persists beyond the age of four years. It may be due to oral motor dysfunction; a deficit of the oral sphincter; inadequate swallowing capacity (e.g. esophageal obstruction); and, less frequently, sialorrhea (Figure 40.2). Drooling is common in neurological conditions (e.g. Alzheimer disease, cerebral palsy, Down syndrome, learning impairment, Parkinsonism, stroke, facial palsy, pseudobulbar palsy, or bulbar palsy).

Drooling may not only be unesthetic (Figure 40.3) but can also affect speech and eating, and lead to functional, social, psychological, and clinical consequences for patients, families, and caregivers. Saliva soils clothing and patients may have perioral skin breakdown and infections, disturbed speech and eating, and can occasionally develop aspiration-related and pulmonary complications.

Diagnosis

Absolute quantification of saliva spill or intraoral pooling by volumetric measurement can help guide treatment; a subjective estimate can be made by counting the bibs or items of clothing soiled each day.

Management

Management options range from conservative therapy to medication, radiation, or surgery, and often a combination is needed. Pharmacological treatment (anti-cholinergic drugs, e.g. atropinics such as hyoscine or ipratropium or adrenergic stimulators, e.g. clonidine) decreases salivation. Botulinum toxin serotype A injections may have a positive outcome. Persistent drooling is managed by redirecting the submandibular duct flow to the back of the mouth; or duct ligation (mainly parotid); or gland removal or neurectomy.

Table 40.2 Investigations used in salivary gland disease.

Procedure	Advantages	Disadvantages	Comments
Blood tests	Simple	Rarely reflect local disease	Can confirm systemic disease (e.g. Sjögren syndrome or rheumatoid arthritis)
CT	Can examine several glands	Expensive; radiation	Useful for investigating space occupying lesions
MRI	Can examine several glands	Expensive	Useful for investigating space occupying lesions
Radiography (plain)	Lower occlusal and oblique lateral or DPT may show submandibular calculi Soft PA film may show parotid calculi	Radiation	Calculi may not be radio-opaque
Salivary gland biopsy	Gives histopathology	Invasive Minor gland biopsy may cause hypoesthesia. Major gland biopsy may result in facial palsy or salivary fistula	Labial gland biopsy is simple and reflects changes in other salivary (and exocrine) glands Major gland biopsy may be diagnostic in localised gland disease Fine needle biopsy may be useful
Sialography	—	Time consuming, crude, insensitive, radiation May cause pain or sialadenitis	Helps eliminate gross structural damage, calculi or stenoses [a]
Sialometry (salivary flow rates)[b]	Simple	Imprecise	Rapid clinical procedure to confirm or refute xerostomia
Scintigraphy and radiosialometry	Measures radionuclide[c] uptake Radiosialometry more quantitative	Radiation taken up by, and rarely damages, thyroid gland	High uptake (hotspots) may reveal tumor Also shows duct patency, gland vascularity and function
Ultrasonography	Non-invasive, inexpensive	User-dependent	Increasingly used

[a] Combined sialography with CT or MRI may be useful particularly in diagnosis and localisation of neoplasms.
[b] Unstimulated whole salivary flow rate (UWSFR) usually used; flow rates < 1.5 ml/15 min are low. Alternatively, stimulate parotid salivary flow with 1 ml 10% citric acid on the tongue or pilocarpine 2.5 mg oral or IV; flow rates < 1 ml/minute may signify reduced salivary function.
[c] Usually technetium pertechnetate.

41

Salivary conditions: Dry mouth

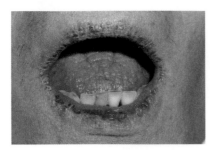

Figure 41.1 Dry mouth: cheilitis.

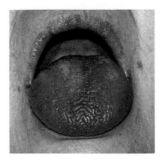

Figure 41.2 Dry mouth: candidosis.

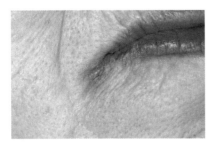

Figure 41.3 Dry mouth: angular stomatitis.

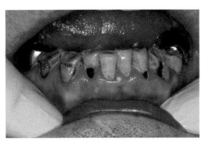

Figure 41.4 Dry mouth: caries.

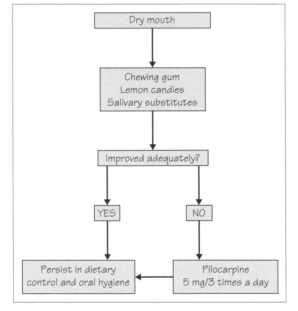

Figure 41.5 Dry mouth management.

Dry mouth (xerostomia; hyposalivation) is a common subjective complaint but objective evidence of hyposalivation is less common, and the complaint is sometimes perceived rather than real.

The main causes are iatrogenic (anticholinergic or sympathomimetic drugs, e.g. tricyclics, phenothiazines and antihistamines; irradiation of salivary glands including incidentally by [131] iodine therapy; cytotoxic agents; or graft-versus-host disease) and non-iatrogenic (dehydration, e.g. uncontrolled diabetes; Sjögren's syndrome; sarcoidosis; HIV disease, rarely cystic fibrosis or salivary gland aplasia) (Table 41.1). Sialosis, calculi or removal of a single major gland rarely cause xerostomia.

Sequelae of hyposalivation include caries, candidosis and ascending sialadenitis.

Diagnosis

Dryness may present because of:
- difficulty eating dry foods (the cracker sign)
- difficulties in controlling dentures in speech and swallowing
- disturbed taste
- soreness, often due to cheilitis (Figure 41.1), candidosis (Figure 41.2) or angular stomatitis (Figure 41.3)
- caries (Figure 41.4)
- sialadenitis.

Mouth dryness may be recognized by:
- the clicking quality of speech as the tongue tends to stick to the palate
- the mucosa tending to stick to a dental mirror
- the mouth may appear dry and glazed; the tongue may develop a characteristic lobulated, usually red, surface with depapillation
- there may be lack of the usual pooling of saliva in the floor of mouth
- thin lines of frothy saliva.

Salivary flow rates will confirm the presence, and degree of xerostomia. Whole saliva collected without stimulation by allowing the patient to dribble into a sterile container over a measured period is now regarded as the best form of sialometry. A value below 1.5 ml/15 mins is regarded as abnormal. Parotid output after stimulation with 10%

citric acid can also be objectively determined using a suction (Lashley or Carlsson-Crittenden) cup over the parotid duct orifice or by cannulation of the duct, but has no advantage. A value below 1.0 ml/min is regarded as abnormal.

Management

It is wise for the patient with dry mouth to use a soft/moist diet and avoid:

- dry foods such as biscuits
- drugs that may produce xerostomia, such as:
  — tricyclics
  — alcohol
  — smoking

Salivary substitutes (mouth wetting agents) may help symptomatically (Figure 41.5). Various are available including:

- water
- methylcellulose
- mucin; artificial saliva

Salivation may be stimulated by using:

- chewing gums (containing sorbitol, not sucrose)
- diabetic sweets
- cholinergic drugs that stimulate salivation (sialogogues), such as pilocarpine or cevimeline; these should be supervised by the specialist

since they may cause other cholinergic effects such as bradycardia, sweating and urge to urinate

- transglossal electrical stimulation

The lips should be protected with petroleum jelly. Complications which should be avoided/treated include:

Dental caries

- Control of dietary sucrose intake.
- Daily use of fluorides (1% sodium fluoride gels or 0.4% stannous fluoride gels) and remineralising casein phosphopeptide-calcium phosphate preparations.

Candidosis

- Dentures should be left out of the mouth at night and stored for a limited period in sodium hypochlorite solution or chlorhexidine.
- An antifungal such as miconazole gel or amphotericin or nystatin ointment should be spread on the denture before re-insertion and a topical antifungal preparation such as nystatin or amphotericin suspension or lozenges used. Fluconazole is also effective.

Bacterial sialadenitis

- Acute sialadenitis needs treating with antibiotics such as amoxicillin/clavulanate or flucloxacillin.

Table 41.1 Causes of dry mouth.

Iatrogenic		Diseases	
Drugs	Drugs with anticholinergic or sympathomimetic effects	**Inflammatory**	Sjögren syndrome
			Sarcoidosis
Procedures	Irradiation	**Infective**	HIV infection
	Chemotherapy		HCV infection
	Bone marrow transplantation		HTLV-1 infection
	Graft-versus-host disease		Other infections
		Other disorders affecting salivary glands	Amyloidosis or other deposits
			Cystic fibrosis
			Dysautonomia
			Ectodermal dysplasia
			Salivary gland aplasia
		Dehydration	Chronic kidney disease
			Diabetes insipidus
			Diabetes mellitus
			Diarrhea and vomiting
			Hyperparathyroidism
			Severe hemorrhage
		Psychogenic	Anxiety states
			Bulimia nervosa
			Depression
			Hypochondriasis

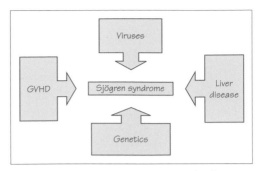

Figure 42.1 Causes of Sjögren syndrome (SS).

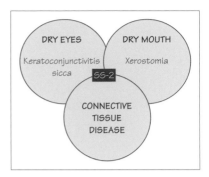

Figure 42.2 Secondary Sjögren syndrome (SS-2).

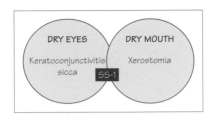

Figure 42.3 Primary Sjögren syndrome (sicca syndrome).

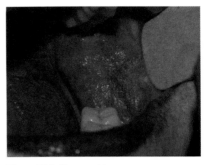

Figure 42.4 Dry mouth.

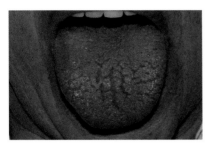

Figure 42.5 Dry mouth.

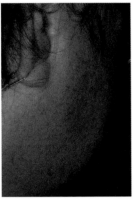

Figure 42.6 Salivary swelling in SS.

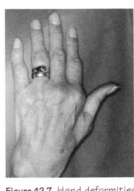

Figure 42.7 Hand deformities in rheumatoid arthritis in SS.

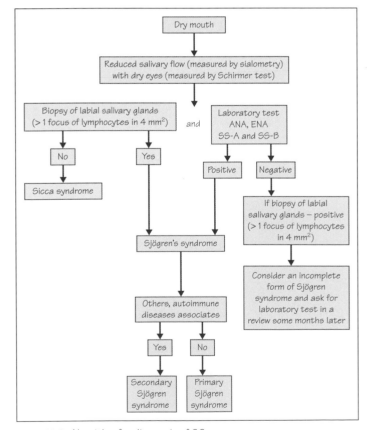

Figure 42.8 Algorithm for diagnosis of SS.

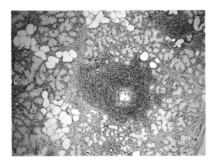

Figure 42.9 Sjögren syndrome focal lymphocytic adenitis.

Definition: The association of dry mouth (xerostomia) and dry eyes (keratoconjunctivitis sicca).

Prevalence (approximate): Uncommon.

Age mainly affected: Older people.

Gender mainly affected: F > M.

Etiopathogenesis: A benign autoimmune inflammatory exocrinopathy (epithelitis) directed against alpha fodrin, a cytoskeletal protein involved in actin binding, with lymphocyte-mediated destruction of salivary, lacrimal and other exocrine glands. Tumor necrosis factor (TNF), interferon (IFN) and B cell activating factor (BAFF) are implicated. A viral etiology, possibly human retrovirus 5 (HRV-5), and a genetic predisposition may be implicated. A SS type of disease may follow HIV, EBV, HCV, or *Helicobacter pylori* infection, or graft-versus-host disease (Figure 42.1).

Most common is *secondary* SS (SS-2) which comprises dry eyes and dry mouth and an autoimmune disease – usually primary biliary cirrhosis or a connective tissue disease such as rheumatoid arthritis (Figure 42.2).

The same features in the absence of systemic autoimmune disease are termed *primary* SS (SS-1 or sicca syndrome) (Figure 42.3).

Diagnostic features

History

Oral: May include:

- xerostomia and sequelae (Chapter 41)
- salivary gland swelling

Extraoral: Eye complaints (e.g. sensations of grittiness, soreness, dryness, blurred vision, discomfort) and Raynaud syndrome (episodic vasospastic attacks, causing blood vessels in fingers and toes to constrict causing pallor and pain), fatigue and epithelitis effects on other organs (kidneys, blood vessels, liver, pancreas, lungs, brain) and immune complex manifestations (arthritis, arthralgia, purpura, rashes, neuropathy, low C4).

Clinical features

Oral: Mouth dryness, recognized by:

- clicking speech
- mucosa tending to stick to dental mirror
- mouth may appear dry and glazed (Figure 42.4); the tongue may become lobulated, red, with depapillation (Figure 42.5)
- lack of pooling of saliva in the floor of mouth
- frothy saliva.

Trigeminal or facial neuropathy may occur.

Sore and red oral mucosa, and angular stomatitis are usually due to candidosis. Dental caries may be severe and difficult to control. Ascending (suppurative) sialadenitis is a hazard.

Salivary swelling is common (Figure 42.6), occasionally massive and associated with lymphadenopathy – pseudolymphoma.

Extraoral: Skin, nose, vaginal and ocular dryness and lacrimal glands swell, plus extraglandular features (Figure 42.7).

Diagnosis is mainly from history and clinical examination. Eyes may be tested for:

- Tears
  - Schirmer test, < 5 mm wetting in five minutes suggests SS
  - tear break-up time reduced
- Eye damage
  - Rose-Bengal 1% staining and slit lamp examination – the staining amount is scored by van Bijsterveld scheme
  Helpful investigations include (Figure 42.8):
- Serum autoantibodies, particularly antinuclear antibodies (ANA) known as SS-A (Ro) and SS-B (La), and rheumatoid factor (RF). SS-A is common in many autoimmune diseases (e.g. systemic lupus erythematosus (SLE) and primary biliary cirrhosis) including SS-2. In contrast, SS-B is more associated with SS-1 (Table 42.1).
- Raised erythrocyte sedimentation rate (ESR) or plasma viscosity.
- Labial gland biopsy (Figure 42.9 and Table 42.2).
- Sialometry – reduced.

Differential diagnosis: Other causes of xerostomia. The diagnostic criteria are shown in Table 42.2. See also Chapter 41.

Management

Artificial tears and saliva can be helpful. An ophthalmological opinion is indicated. Drugs to control underlying autoimmune disease (e.g. ciclosporin, anti-cytokines (against TNF, interferon, BAFF) and anti-B cell monoclonal antibodies against CD20 (rituximab) and CD22 (epratuzumab)) are experimental only.

Prognosis

There is low mortality but lymphoid malignancy develops in ~ 5%, particularly in patients with severe SS, purpura, low C4 and mixed monoclonal cryoglobulinemia.

Table 42.1 Sjögren syndrome: Main serum autoantibodies.

Autoantibody	SS-1	SS-2
SS-A	+	++
SS-B	++	+
RF	++	+++

Table 42.2 Diagnostic criteria (American-European) for Sjögren syndrome.

I **Ocular symptoms**	A positive response to at least one of the following questions:	(1) Have you had daily ocular symptoms or persistent, troublesome dry eyes for more than three months? (2) Do you have a recurrent sensation of sand or gravel in the eyes? (3) Do you use tear substitutes more than 3 times a day?
II **Oral symptoms**	A positive response to at least one of the following questions:	(1) Have you had a daily feeling of dry mouth for more than 3 months? (2) Have you had recurrently or persistently swollen salivary glands as an adult? (3) Do you frequently drink liquids to aid in swallowing dry food?
III **Ocular signs**	That is, objective evidence of ocular involvement defined as a positive result for at least one of:	(1) Schirmer test, performed without anesthesia (< 5 mm in 5 minutes). (2) Rose-Bengal score or other ocular dye score (> 4 according to van Bijsterveld's scoring system).
IV **Histopathology**	In minor salivary glands (obtained through normal-appearing mucosa).	Focal lymphocytic sialadenitis evaluated by an expert histopathologist, with a focus score > 1, defined as a number of lymphocytic foci (which are adjacent to normal-appearing mucous acini and contain more than 50 lymphocytes) per 4 mm^2 of glandular tissue.
V **Salivary gland involvement**	Objective evidence of salivary gland involvement, defined by a positive result for one of the following:	(1) Unstimulated whole salivary flow ≤ 1.5 ml in 15 minutes. (2) Parotid sialography showing the presence of ductal sialectasis (punctate, cavitary or destructive pattern) without evidence of obstruction in the major ducts. (3) Salivary scintigraphy showing delayed uptake, reduced concentration and/or delayed excretion of tracer.
VI **Autoantibodies**	Presence in the serum of the following autoantibodies:	Antibodies to Ro (SS-A) or La (SS-B) antigens, or both.

43

Salivary conditions: Sialolithiasis, sialadenitis

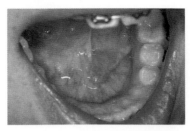

Figure 43.1a Sialolithiasis.

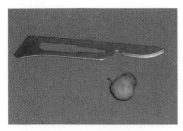

Figure 43.1b Sialolithiasis.

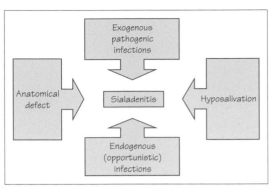

Figure 43.2 Sialadenitis: causes.

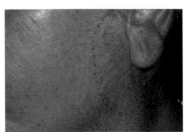

Figure 43.3 Sialadenitis.

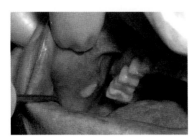

Figure 43.4 Sialadenitis showing pus from Stensen duct.

Sialolithiasis

Definition: Calculus, usually in a salivary duct.
  Prevalence (approximate): Uncommon.
  Age mainly affected: Older adults.
  Gender mainly affected: M = F.
  Etiopathogenesis: Possibly salivary stasis.

Diagnostic features
History
Oral: Symptomless, or pain/swelling related to meals.

Clinical features
Oral: Salivary calculi (sialoliths):
- usually affect the submandibular duct (Figures 43.1a and 43.1b)
- are usually yellow or white and can sometimes be seen in the duct
- may be palpable
- are commonly radiopaque
  Calculi are even less common in the parotid and then are typically radiolucent, and are rare in minor glands. Calculi may lead to sialadenitis.
  Differential diagnosis: Other causes of salivary gland swelling.
  Imaging: Sialography if necessary (Figure 5.8).

Management
Surgical, endoscopic or lithotripsy removal of obstruction.

Prognosis
Good.

Sialadenitis
Sialadenitis may arise from a number of causes (Figure 43.2).

Sialadenitis: Acute viral (mumps)

Definition: An acute infectious viral infection of salivary glands.
  Prevalence (approximate): Common.
  Age mainly affected: Children.
  Gender mainly affected: M = F.
  Etiopathogenesis: Usually infection with the mumps virus (an RNA paramyxovirus). Transmission of classical mumps is by direct contact or by droplet spread from saliva.
  Rarely, other viruses (e.g. Coxsackie, ECHO, EBV, CMV, HCV or HIV) cause similar syndromes.

Diagnostic features
History
Oral: Swollen salivary glands.
  Extraoral: Headache, malaise, anorexia.
  Clinical features: An incubation period of 2–3 weeks elapses before clinical features appear, and up to 30% are subclinical.
  Oral: Parotitis and trismus. Acute onset of painful, usually bilaterally, enlarged parotids, although in the early stages only one parotid gland may appear to be involved (Figure 43.3). The submandibular glands may also be affected.
  The skin over the affected glands appears normal, as does the saliva – features which help distinguish from acute bacterial sialadenitis.
  Extraoral: May include:
- fever
- inflammation of testes (orchitis) or ovaries (oophoritis); ensuing infertility is rare
- pancreatitis
- meningitis or meningoencephalitis
- deafness – rare but profound.

Diagnosis is clinical but confirmation, if needed, is by demonstrating a four-fold rise in serum antibody titers between acute and convalescent serum (taken three weeks later); raised levels of serum amylases, or lipases, or mumps virus PCR or nested polymerase chain reaction.

Management
Mumps is a notifiable disease in the UK (the Proper Officer of the local authority must be notified).

No specific antiviral agents are available. Treatment is symptomatic. MMR vaccine protects against mumps, measles and rubella.

Prognosis
Good.

Sialadenitis: Acute bacterial ascending
Definition: Sialadenitis due to bacterial infection ascending from the oral cavity.

Prevalence (approximate): Rare.

Age mainly affected: Older adults.

Gender mainly affected: M = F.

Etiopathogenesis: The organisms most commonly isolated in ascending sialadenitis are *Streptococcus viridans* and *Staphylococcus aureus* (often penicillin-resistant). The parotid glands are most commonly affected, and it may be seen:
- after radiotherapy to the head and neck
- in Sjögren syndrome
- occasionally following gastrointestinal surgery, because of dehydration and dry mouth
- rarely in otherwise apparently healthy patients, when it is usually due to salivary abnormalities such as calculi, mucus plugs and duct strictures.

Diagnostic features
History
Oral: Painful salivary gland swelling.

Extraoral: +/− trismus, lymphadenitis and fever.

Clinical features
Oral: Acute parotitis typically presents with:
- painful and tender enlargement of one gland only
- the overlying skin possibly reddened
- pus exuding from, or milked from, the parotid duct orifice (Figure 43.4)
- trismus

If the infection localizes as a parotid abscess, it may point externally through the overlying skin or, rarely, into the external acoustic meatus.

Extraoral: Cervical lymphadenopathy, pyrexia.

Differential diagnosis
The diagnosis is essentially clinical but pus should be sent for culture and sensitivity testing.

Management
- Analgesia and prompt therapy with amoxicillin (flucloxacillin or amoxicillin/clavulanate if staphylococcus and not allergic to penicillin; erythromycin or azithromycin in penicillin allergy).
- Surgical drainage is needed where there is fluctuation.
- Hydration.
- Salivation should be stimulated by chewing gum or use of sialogogues.

Prognosis
Good.

Sialadenitis: Chronic bacterial
Definition: Chronic salivary gland infection.

Prevalence (approximate): Rare.

Age mainly affected: Older adults.

Gender mainly affected: M = F.

Etiopathogenesis: May develop after salivary calculus formation or acute sialadenitis, particularly if inappropriate antibiotics are used, or predisposing factors not eliminated. Serous acini atrophy when salivary outflow is chronically obstructed, further reducing saliva secretion.

Diagnostic features
History
Oral: Affected gland is chronically swollen.

Clinical features
Oral: Single swollen, firm, non-tender salivary gland.

Extraoral: No systemic features of infection.

Differential diagnosis: Calculus, neoplasm.

Diagnosis is from clinical features, and imaging (radiography, MRI, ultrasonography).

Management
Surgical excision is often needed.

Prognosis
Good.

Sialadenitis: Recurrent parotitis of childhood
Definition: Repeated parotitis and sialectasis in a child, associated with a sialographic pattern of sialectasis.

Prevalence (approximate): Uncommon.

Age mainly affected: Usually begins in pre-school children.

Gender mainly affected: M > F.

Etiopathogenesis: Congenital or autoimmune duct defects.

Diagnostic features
History
Oral: Little pain. Intermittent, unilateral parotid swelling which lasts < 3 weeks with spontaneous regression. It may occur simultaneously or alternately contra-laterally.

Extraoral: Occasional fever.

Clinical features
Oral: Parotid swelling.

Differential diagnosis: Sjögren syndrome.

Diagnosis is mainly on clinical grounds but serum anti-SS-A and SS-B antibodies are indicated to exclude Sjögren syndrome, and imaging with ultrasonography and CT scan or sialography showing sialectasis is confirmatory.

Management
Medical: Episodes are managed with sialogogues, glandular massage, and duct probing to promote ductal lavage. No specific treatment is available. Antibiotics and corticosteroids are limited in value; surgery is unnecessary.

Prognosis
Often remits around puberty.

44

Salivary conditions: Neoplasms

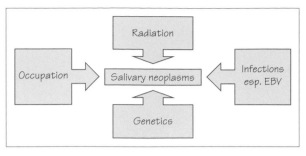

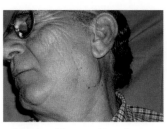

Figure 44.1 Salivary neoplasms; aetiology.

Figure 44.2 Pleomorphic salivary adenoma.

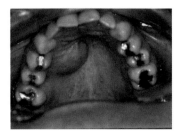

Figure 44.3 Pleomorphic salivary adenoma.

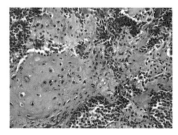

Figure 44.4 Pleomorphic salivary adenoma.

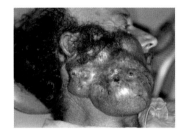

Figure 44.5 Giant malignant pleomorphic adenoma.

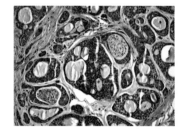

Figure 44.6 Cribiform adenoid cystic carcinoma with perineural invasion.

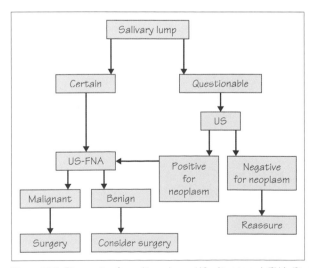

Figure 44.7 Diagnosis of a salivary lump. US-ultrasound; FNA-Fine Needle Aspiration biopsy.

Definition: Neoplasms affect major or minor salivary glands and can be benign or malignant.

Prevalence (approximate): 1 per 100,000.

Age mainly affected: Older adults.

Gender mainly affected: F > M for benign, but F = M for malignant tumors.

Etiopathogenesis: There may be an association with breast cancer. Irradiation is implicated in some neoplasms but speculation that mobile (cell) telephone electromagnetic fields increase the risk has not been confirmed. Other risk factors include tobacco smoking in Warthin tumor; EBV in some tumors (Figure 44.1), HIV/AIDS and occupations involving wood dust exposure.

Pathogenesis involves p53 tumor-suppressor gene and oncogenes. For example, pleomorphic salivary adenoma (PSAs) often have allelic loss on chromosome 12 where HMGIC (high-mobility group protein isoform I-C – implicated in control of cell proliferation and development) is located, and changes on chromosome 8 where PLAG1 (pleomorphic adenoma gene 1) is involved. High levels of nitric oxide synthase and vascular endothelial growth factor (VEGF) correlate with tumor stage, size, invasion, recurrence, metastases, poor prognosis, and aggression.

Diagnostic features

History

Oral: Symptomless, or swelling and/or pain. Slow gradual gland enlargement suggests a benign process. Pain or facial nerve palsy raise suspicions of carcinoma.

Clinical features: Any salivary swelling, especially if localized, firm and persistent, may be neoplastic.

Tumors of major salivary glands mostly:
• present as unilateral swelling
• affect the parotid (Figure 44.2)
• are benign
• are PSAs or Warthin tumor.

The "rule of nines" is that nine out of ten tumors affect the parotid, nine out of ten are benign, and nine out of ten are PSAs.

Tumors of intraoral salivary glands are less common than in major glands but more frequently malignant, and are mostly:
• PSAs (but adenoid cystic carcinoma and mucoepidermoid carcinoma are relatively more common than in major glands)
• unilateral
• seen most commonly as a firm, well-circumscribed, smooth swelling on the posterior palate (Figure 44.3) (occasionally buccal mucosa or upper lip; rarely, tongue or lower lip).

Most tumors in the:
• parotid – are PSAs and benign
• lips – are in the upper lip and benign (PSAs or canalicular adenomas)
• submandibular – are PSAs and benign but one-half are malignant
• sublingual gland – are malignant
• tongue – are malignant, especially adenoid cystic carcinoma.

Benign neoplasms (adenomas)

PSA (mixed tumor) is:
• the most common tumor
• usually solitary
• usually slow-growing
• a lobulated, rubbery swelling with normal overlying skin or mucosa, but a bluish appearance if intra-oral
• in intimate relationship with the facial nerve and poorly encapsulated, if in the parotid

Histopathology shows mixed epithelial and mesenchymal cell components, the latter often having a myxofibrous appearance and sometimes chondromatous differentiation (Figure 44.4).

Warthin tumor is the next most common tumor, found almost exclusively in the parotids, bilaterally in 10%, and more common in men. Typically, it is in the gland tail and an encapsulated, smooth, round lesion with multiple communicating cysts. It is a benign monomorphic tumor with lymphoid tissue covered by epithelium (adenolymphoma; papillary cystadenoma lymphomatosum).

Canalicular adenoma is typically seen in older females, 95% in the upper lip, others in the buccal mucosa. It contains cords of columnar or cuboidal cells with basophilic nuclei.

Oncocytoma (oxyphilic adenoma) is a rare neoplasm found only in the parotid, and mainly in older people.

Malignant neoplasms

Malignant tumors are of variable malignancy, and most metastasize late (Figure 44.5) and include:
• *Mucoepidermoid carcinoma*: One of the more common tumors, usually slow-growing, and of low-grade malignancy. It presents as a painless, slow-growing firm or hard mass. It is unencapsulated, contains squamous, mucus-secreting, and intermediate cells and has a good prognosis for low-grade, and poor prognosis for high-grade tumors.
• *Adenoid cystic carcinoma* (cylindroma): Slow-growing, malignant and infiltrates perineurally and metastasizes mainly distantly, not in regional lymph nodes. It has a "Swiss cheese" histopathological appearance (Figure 44.6).
• *Polymorphous low-grade carcinoma*: Slow-growing, malignant, seen in minor glands in older females, and rarely metastasizes.
• *Acinic cell carcinoma*: Rare and often low-grade malignancy.
• *Carcinoma in PSA*: Rare.
• *Salivary duct carcinoma*: Rare, involves mainly the parotid, and is aggressive, with an unfavorable prognosis.

Differential diagnosis: From other causes of salivary swelling.

Early detection improves prognosis.
• MRI, CT and ultrasonography are most commonly used. Gadolinium-enhanced dynamic MRI may differentiate PSAs and Warthin tumors from malignancies.
• F-18 fluorodeoxyglucose (FDG)-PET (Positron Emission Tomography) can detect lymph node and distant metastases. It is most useful when combined with CT. Tc-99m (Technetium-99m) pertechnetate scintigraphy can help diagnose Warthin tumors with correlation between size and Tc-99m uptake.
• Sialography may reveal an obvious filling defect or gland displacement.
• Pre-operative fine needle aspiration (FNA) biopsy, and core needle biopsy (larger needle), particularly if ultrasound (US) or CT guided, is useful in major glands (Figure 44.7), having a high tumor detection rate, especially in the submandibular gland.
• The diagnosis may best be firmly established by open biopsy, often carried out at the definitive operation.

Management

Benign parotid tumors: Superficial or, when necessary, total parotidectomy. Malignant tumors: Wide local resection, adjuvant radiotherapy.

Extreme care is necessary to avoid facial nerve damage.

Prognosis

Varies dependent on tumor type, location and treatment.

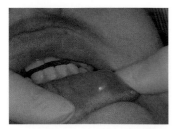

Figure 45.1 Mucocele.

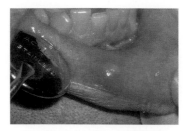

Figure 45.2 Mucocele.

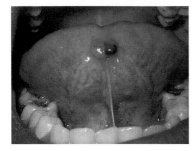

Figure 45.3 Mucocele.

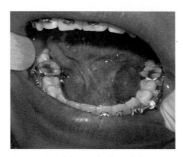

Figure 45.4 Mucocele (ranula).

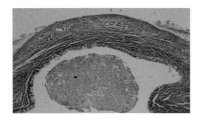

Figure 45.5 Retention cyst of minor salivary gland.

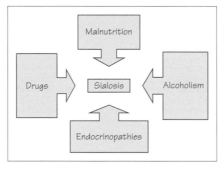

Figure 45.6 Sialosis: causes.

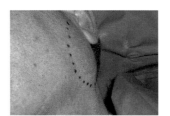

Figure 45.7 Sialosis.

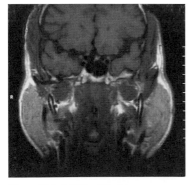

Figure 45.8 MRI in sialosis.

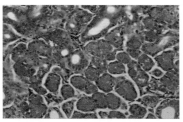

Figure 45.9 Histopathology in sialosis showing acinar hypertrophy.

Mucoceles (mucous cyst; mucus extravasation phenomenon; myxoid cyst)

Definition: A mucus-filled cyst.

Prevalence (approximate): Common.

Age mainly affected: Young adults/children.

Gender mainly affected: M > F.

Etiopathogenesis; Most mucus-filled cysts are *mucoceles* (90–95%) – extravasation mucoceles due to ductal damage; most are seen in the lower labial mucosa or on the lower lip, presumably resulting from trauma from lip-biting, resulting from the escape of mucus from a damaged minor salivary gland duct into the lamina propria.

Occasionally, mucus-filled cysts are *mucus retention cysts* – mucus is retained within a salivary gland or duct; most are seen in the upper lip or sublingually (ranula).

Rarely, mucus extravasates intra- or subepithelially – *superficial mucoceles*, seen mainly in lichen planus; palatal lesions are most common.

Multiple *lymphoepithelial cysts* may be seen in major salivary glands in HIV disease and on the lateral border of tongue/floor of mouth.

Diagnostic features

History

Oral: A single, painless, dome-shaped, translucent, whitish blue papule or nodule which ruptures easily to release viscid salty mucus, but frequently recurs.

Clinical features

Oral: Usually a single, fluctuant dome-shaped, translucent, whitish blue swelling, papule or nodule, mostly inside lower lip, sometimes buccal mucosa, palate or ventrum of tongue/floor of mouth (Figures 45.1–45.4). Range from 1 mm to 1 cm or more in diameter.

Differential diagnosis: From a salivary gland tumor with cystic change, especially when in the upper lip and, in endemic regions, from cysticercosis (in taeniasis).

Investigations

Biopsy/histopathology: Shows mucus spilling out into the tissues from the damaged duct evoking an acute inflammatory reaction with vascular hyperemia, fibrin exudation and granulation tissue formation (Figure 45.5). Initially the lesion is diffuse, and may be dismissed microscopically as an acute inflammatory lesion or merely granulation tissue. However, under higher power there are foamy macrophages, which are macrophages that have ingested mucus (mucinophages). At a later stage there is much less inflammation in the surrounding tissues because the mucocele is walled off by fibrous tissue. The cyst is lined by mucus-containing macrophages which in some cases look like epithelial cells. Some mucoceles are so superficial that they produce a subepithelial or intraepithelial blister and can be mistaken microscopically for vesiculo-bullous lesions such as mucous membrane pemphigoid and pemphigus vulgaris.

Mucocele and mucous retention cysts differ somewhat clinically and microscopically. Mucous retention cysts are typically non-inflamed and lined by attenuated epithelium which may be columnar or sometimes stratified. It is important to examine such lesions carefully, because salivary gland tumors, both benign and malignant, can present with a significant cystic component. The tumor may only be a small area of mural thickening in a cyst and is easy to miss. Therefore, it is essential to examine the whole specimen and not just assume that the lesion is a cyst.

Management

Medical: If asymptomatic and small, observe.

Surgical: The cysts can be excised but they also respond well to cryosurgery, using a single freeze-thaw cycle (but then histology is lost).

Prognosis

Good. Recurrences are rare, possibly if the damaged gland persists.

Sialosis (sialadenosis)

Definition: Bilaterally, symmetrical painless enlargement of salivary glands.

Prevalence (approximate): Uncommon.

Age mainly affected: Adults.

Gender mainly affected: M > F.

Etiopathogenesis: Dysregulation of the autonomic innervation of the salivary glands is the unifying factor. The main causes include (Figure 45.6):

- Alcoholism
  - alcohol abuse with or without accompanying liver cirrhosis
- Endocrine conditions
  - diabetes mellitus
  - acromegaly
  - thyroid disease
  - pregnancy
- Nutritional disorders
  - anorexia nervosa
  - bulimia
  - cystic fibrosis with malnutrition
- Drugs
  - sympathomimetic drugs such as isoprenaline.

Diagnostic features

History

Oral: Persistent painless salivary swellings.

Extraoral: Depends on cause.

Clinical features

Oral: Salivary gland swelling; soft, painless and usually bilateral (usually the parotids), no xerostomia, no trismus (Figure 45.7).

Extraoral: No fever.

Differential diagnosis: Sjögren's syndrome, sarcoidosis, benign lymphoepithelial lesion, sialadenitis, neoplasms, deposits.

Investigations

The diagnosis of sialosis is one of exclusion, based mainly on history and clinical examination.

Salivary gland function is normal: MRI (Figure 45.8), sialography and ultrasonography usually show enlarged but normal glands. Salivary biopsy is rarely indicated (Figure 45.9).

Sialochemistry may show raised potassium and calcium levels which would not be present in salivary enlargement due to other causes. Blood examination for raised glucose levels, possibly growth hormone levels, or abnormal liver function may point to an underlying cause.

Management

No specific treatment is available but sialosis may resolve when causal factors resolve (alcohol intake is reduced, glucose control instituted or eating disorders remit).

Prognosis

Good.

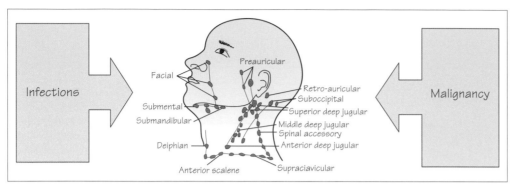

Figure 46.1 Cervical lymphadenopathy: causes.

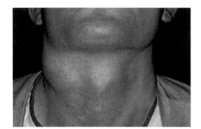

Figure 46.2 Lymphadenitis.

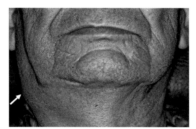

Figure 46.3a Lymph node metastasis.

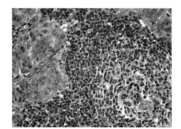

Figure 46.3b Metastasis from squamous carcinoma 40 ×.

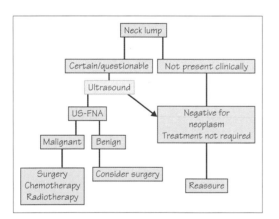

Figure 46.4a Diagnosis of neck lumps. US–FNA, ultrasound and fine needle aspiration biopsy.

Table 46.1 Main causes of swelling in the neck.

Lymph nodes	Skin, muscle or other soft tissue	Thyroid	Salivary glands	Other tissues
Connective tissue disease	Any soft tissue inflammation, cyst or neoplasm	Ectopic thyroid	See Table 40.1	Branchial cyst
Drugs (e.g. phenytoin)				
Granulomatous diseases	Dermoid cyst	Thyroglossal cyst		Carotid body tumors or
Infections	Hematoma	Thyroid tumors		aneurysms
Neoplasms	Infections	or goitre		Cystic
	Edema			hygroma
	"Plunging" ranula			Pharyngeal
	Surgical emphysema			pouch

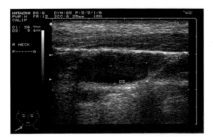

Figure 46.4b Ultrasound of a large jugulo-digastric lymph node. Courtesy of J. Brown, C. Scully and Private Dentistry.

Discrete swellings in the neck

These commonly arise in cervical lymph nodes but may occasionally arise elsewhere (Table 46.1).

There are approximately 300 cervical lymph nodes (about one-third of the body's lymphoid tissue). Lymphadenopathy, the term meaning "disease of lymph nodes" is often used synonymously with "swollen/enlarged lymph nodes"; it generally signifies pathology in the local area of drainage (Table 46.2), usually an infection, when the term "lymphadenitis" is appropriate, but sometimes it is caused by malignancy (Figure 46.1).

Cervical lymphadenopathy

Lymphadenitis is the most common cause of cervical lymphadenopathy, and of a swelling in the neck (Figure 46.2).

Infection

Cervical lymphadenitis in isolation usually arises because of an immune response to an infectious agent. The nodes are then often firm, discrete and tender, but are mobile. The responsible focus can usually be found in the drainage area (Table 46.2). Any bacterial infection, such as a dental abscess, pericoronitis, sinusitis, or a nasal abscess, can be responsible, as can viral or other local infections. Occasionally, the source cannot be identified despite a careful search. For example, children (especially those of African heritage) occasionally develop a *Staphylococcus aureus* lymphadenitis, usually of a submandibular lymph node, in the absence of any obvious portal of infection. Such infections should be treated with antibiotics – usually flucloxacillin or amoxicillin/clavulanate. If the lesion is pointing, drainage is needed. A similar problem may arise due to mycobacteria. Cervical mycobacterial lymphadenitis (scrofula) has increased and may be the manifestation of systemic tuberculosis (TB) or a unique clinical entity localized to neck. TB lymphadenitis is not uncommon among patients from the developing world and people on peritoneal dialysis. A unilateral single or multiple painless lump, mostly located in posterior cervical or supraclavicular region can occur. It remains a diagnostic and therapeutic challenge because it mimics other pathologic processes and yields inconsistent physical and laboratory findings.

A thorough history and physical examination, tuberculin test, staining for acid fast bacilli, and radiologic examination are indicated by fine needle aspiration (FNA) biopsy of the cervical lymph nodes; this is the most reliable diagnostic method, since few patients have positive chest radiographs, tuberculin skin test, or culture for mycobacteria. It is important to differentiate tuberculous from nontuberculous mycobacterial cervical lymphadenitis because tuberculous adenitis is best treated as a systemic disease with antituberculosis medication, while infections with atypical mycobacteria can be treated as local infections and are often amenable to surgical therapy.

Syphilis and brucellosis can also cause cervical lymphadenopathy. Cat-scratch disease on the face or head, caused by *Bartonella henselae* or *Bartonella clarridgeiae* may cause lymphadenitis.

Viral upper respiratory (e.g. common cold or tonsillitis) or oral infections (e.g. those that also produce ulcers) are a common cause of cervical lymphadenitis. Parasitic infections are a rare cause but toxoplasmosis may cause posterior cervical lymphadenopathy.

Malignant disease

Enlargement of cervical lymph nodes in isolation may occur when there is reactive hyperplasia to a malignant tumor in the drainage area, or metastatic infiltration (Figures 46.3a and b). Malignant disease in a node may cause it to feel enlarged and distinctly hard, and it may become bound down to adjacent tissues ("fixed"); it may not be discrete, and may even, in advanced cases, ulcerate through the skin. Neoplasms that usually metastasize to cervical lymph nodes are:

- Oral and antral carcinoma.
- Tonsillar carcinoma: Unsuspected tonsillar cancer is the commonest cause of a cervical node metastasis of unidentified origin. Blind tonsillar biopsy may reveal occult malignancy.
- Nasopharyngeal and nasal carcinoma: Clinically unsuspected nasopharyngeal cancer is a common cause of a cervical node metastasis of unidentified origin. Blind nasopharyngeal biopsy, particularly the fossa of Rosenmüller, may reveal occult malignancy.
- Thyroid tumors.
- Salivary tumors.
- Skin tumors.
- Other metastatic neoplasms (lymphoid and others).
- More than 25% of malignant tumors in children occur in the head and neck, and the cervical lymph nodes are the most common site of presentation.

Ultrasound-guided FNA can be helpful in diagnosis (Figures 46.4a and b).

Unexplained lymphadenopathy

Children sometimes have cervical (or even generalized lymphadenopathy), without an evident cause. Adults may also, but then latent malignant causes are always a concern. One study showed a 0.6% annual incidence of unexplained lymphadenopathy in the general population. Nevertheless, every effort should be made to elicit the cause of lymphadenopathy.

Diffuse swelling of the neck

This may be caused by infection, fluid accumulation (e.g. edema, hematoma, or surgical emphysema (typically the accidental introduction of air into the tissues from dental air-rotor or 3-in-1 syringe)) or malignant infiltration.

Table 46.2 Cervical lymph nodes and their drainage areas.

Lymph nodes	Main drainage areas
Submental	Lower lip, floor of mouth, teeth, sublingual salivary gland, tip of tongue, cheek
Submandibular	Tongue, submandibular gland, lips and mouth
Jugulodigastric (tonsillar)	Tongue, tonsil, pinna, parotid
Posterior cervical	Scalp and neck, cervical and axillary nodes
Suboccipital	Scalp and head
Preauricular	Eyelids, conjunctivae, temporal region, pinna
Postauricular	External auditory meatus, pinna, scalp

47

Neck swelling: Cervical lymphadenopathy in generalized lymphadenopathy

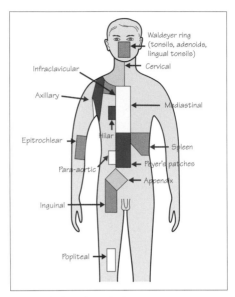

Figure 47.1 Lymphoreticular system.

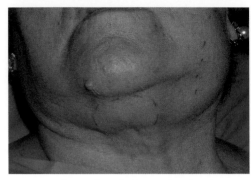

Figure 47.2 Cervical lymphadenopathy – lymphoma.

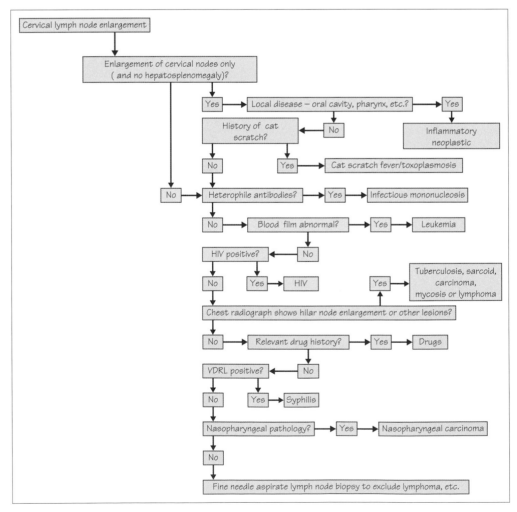

Figure 47.3 Diagnosis in cervical lymphadenopathy.

When two or more lymph node groups are enlarged, the term "generalized lymphadenopathy" is used. This often results from conditions affecting the wider lymphoreticular system (e.g. liver, spleen and lymph nodes in axillary, inguinal, lung hilar area, abdominal wall) (Figure 47.1), especially systemic infections or malignant disease. Causes are decribed below.

Systemic infections

- *Viral* exanthemata (infections mainly in children that produce rashes, e.g. chickenpox, measles, rubella); systemic viral infections, such as glandular fever syndromes (caused by Epstein–Barr virus (EBV), cytomegalovirus (CMV), human herpesvirus 6, and HIV/AIDS), and virus-associated hemophagocytic syndrome (VAHS: a rare consequence of infection with some herpesviruses that damage blood cells).
- *Bacterial* infections, such as tuberculosis, brucellosis and syphilis.
- *Deep mycoses*: paracoccidioidomycosis.
- *Parasitic* infections: Leishmaniasis (*Leishmania infantum/chagasi, L. braziliensis* or *L. tropica* contracted from sand flies); toxoplasmosis (*Toxoplasma gondii*, contracted from cats or their feces often causing posterior cervical lymphadenopathy); and trypanosomiasis (*Trypanosoma brucei*; transmitted by tsetse flies).

Inflammatory disorders (not known to be infective)

- *Connective tissue diseases* (e.g. rheumatoid arthritis, systemic lupus erythematosus).
- *Granulomatous diseases* (e.g. Crohn disease, orofacial granulomatosis, sarcoidosis). Sarcoidosis is a multi-system granulomatous disorder, seen most commonly in Afro-Caribbean young adult females in Northern Europe. The cause of sarcoidosis is unclear but *Propionobacterium acnes*, *P. granulosum* and *Mycobacterium tuberculosis* have been implicated. Sarcoidosis is protean in its manifestations and can involve virtually any tissue, especially hilar lymph nodes, and sometimes other nodes such as cervical nodes.
- *Mucocutaneous lymph node syndrome* (Kawasaki disease) is a vasculitis in children causing fever, rash, red or swollen hands or feet, conjunctivitis, dry and cracked lips, sore red throat or tongue, and cervical lymphadenopathy. May be cardiac complications.

Neoplastic causes

- *Lymphoreticular neoplasms* (e.g. lymphomas, leukemias, lymphomatoid granulomatosis and histiocytoses) usually cause enlargement of many or all lymph nodes (Figure 47.2) and the whole reticuloendothelial system – in many there is generalized lymphadenopathy and hepatosplenomegaly (enlarged liver and spleen).
- *Lymphomatoid granulomatosis*: An EBV-associated and chemotherapy-resistant disorder, with polymorphic lymphoid infiltrates involving lung, skin, and central nervous system.
- *Langerhans cell histiocytosis* (Chapter 56).
- *Rosai-Dorfman disease*: A rare, non-neoplastic histiocytosis characterized by painless, massive cervical lymphadenopathy.
- *Secondary neoplasms* (e.g. metastases, neuroblastoma). During the first six years of life, neuroblastoma and leukemia are the most common

tumors associated with cervical lymphadenopathy, followed by rhabdomyosarcoma and non-Hodgkin lymphoma.

Rare causes of cervical metastases include metastases from the stomach or even testicular tumors to the lower cervical nodes, especially the supraclavicular nodes. Virchow node (Troisier's sign) is a firm, supraclavicular node, usually on the left side in an adult, secondary to primary neoplasm in the thorax or abdomen – usually lymphoma, thoracic or retroperitoneal cancer. Right supraclavicular lymph node enlargement can be due to lung, retroperitoneal or gastrointestinal cancer.

Drugs

- *Drug-induced hypersensitivity syndrome* (DIHS) may manifest with a glandular fever-like syndrome (fever, rash, cervical lymphadenopathy, raised white cell count with atypical lymphocytes, and liver dysfunction). Drugs implicated include anticonvulsants such as carbamazepine and phenytoin, isoniazid and sulfonamides. Some cases are associated with reactivation of HHV-6 or other herpesvirus.

Others

- *Castleman disease* (CD): Also called angiofollicular or giant lymph node hyperplasia and angiomatous lymphoid hamartoma, this is probably due to interleukin-6 hypersecretion. Multicentric CD involves growths at multiple sites and about 50% is caused by KSHV (Kaposi sarcoma herpes virus); there is no standard agreed therapy. Unicentric CD involves only a single node; removal of the enlarged node is curative.
- *Chronic granulomatous disease*: A rare genetic leukocyte defect in which neutrophils and macrophages fail to kill catalase-positive bacteria such as staphylococci. Patients thus suffer recurrent pyogenic infections and develop suppurating cervical lymph nodes showing granulomas on biopsy.
- *Kikuchi disease*: A self-limiting, benign necrotizing lymphadenitis, characterized by fever, neutropenia and cervical lymphadenopathy, seen mainly in young women of Asian descent. The cause is unclear but may be viral.

Diagnosis in generalized lymphadenopathy

The history may elicit relevant features (e.g. fever, night sweats, or weight loss). Physical examination, particularly directed at palpating axillary and inguinal lymph nodes, liver and spleen, and imaging of chest and abdomen may be indicated (to detect lymphadenopathy in chest hilar lymph nodes or abdominal para-aortic nodes), as well as blood tests to exclude infections, leukemias and sarcoidosis (Figure 47.3).

For patients without initial infective symptoms, nodal biopsy is recommended if lymphadenopathy persists beyond 4–6 weeks; if it continues to enlarge; if it is > 3 cm; or if there is supraclavicular lymphadenopathy or concomitant constitutional symptoms (e.g. weight loss or night sweat). Ultrasound or CT can help. Fine needle aspiration (FNA) biopsy is a minimally invasive method for obtaining a tissue sample from a node, but excisional biopsy may be required to provide a definitive diagnosis.

If generalized lymphadenopathy persists for some time, even when no explanation can be found, it is termed "persistent generalized lymphadenopathy" (PGL).

48

Neurological conditions: Bell palsy, and trigeminal sensory loss

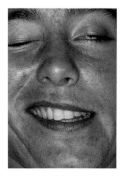

Figure 48.1 Bell palsy of left side.

Table 48.1 Main causes of facial palsy.

Intracranial	Extracerebral in the region of the			Myopathies
	Temporal bone	Middle ear	Parotid	
Cerebral tumor, Connective tissue disorders Crohn's disease Diabetes mellitus Multiple sclerosis Stroke	Ramsay–Hunt syndrome	Cholesteatoma (destructive and expanding keratinizing squamous epithelium in middle ear) Malignancy Mastoiditis	Bell palsy Parotid malignancy Melkersson-Rosenthal syndrome Sarcoidosis (Heerfordt syndrome) Trauma to facial nerve or branches	Myasthenia gravis

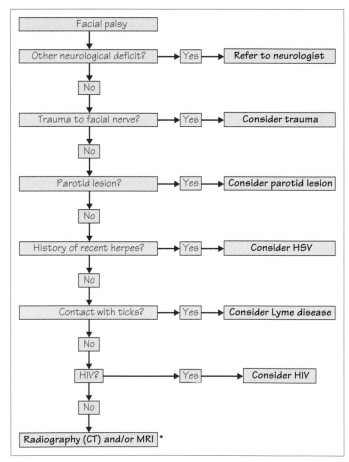

Figure 48.2 Diagnosis of facial palsy. *Brain/skull base.

Box 48.1 Causes of orofacial sensory loss.

Extracranial
Benign tumors
Malignant neoplasms
Osteomyelitis
Trauma (facial or dental)
Intracranial
Amyloidosis
Aneurysms
Cerebrovascular disease
Connective tissue diseases
Diabetes mellitus
HIV/AIDS
Malignant disease
Multiple sclerosis
Sarcoidosis
Sickle cell anemia
Syphilis
Trauma
Vasculitis

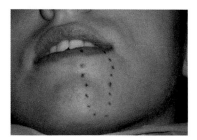

Figure 48.3 Mental nerve sensory loss.

Bell palsy

Definition: An acute lower motor neurone paralysis (palsy) of the face, representing about 50% of all facial palsies (Table 48.1).

Prevalence (approximate): 1 per 10,000.

Age mainly affected: Young adult.

Gender mainly affected: M = F.

Etiopathogenesis: No local or systemic cause can be identified in Bell palsy (it is idiopathic). There is pressure from inflammation and edema on the facial nerve, usually in the stylomastoid canal, with demyelination. Similar lesions are associated:
- Usually with herpes simplex virus (HSV).
- Rarely with another viral infection such as another herpesvirus, HIV or human T lymphotropic virus 1 (HTLV-1); or a bacterium such as in otitis media or *Borrelia burgdorferi* infection (Lyme disease, contracted from the bite of a deer tick).
- Occasionally with pregnancy, hypertension, diabetes, lymphoma, multiple sclerosis or chronic granulomatous disorders (e.g. Crohn disease or orofacial granulomatosis, when the association is often the Melkersson-Rosenthal syndrome (Chapter 27)).

Diagnostic features

History

Oral: Acute paralysis appears over a few hours, maximal within 48 hours. Pain around the ear or jaw may precede palsy by a day or two. May be twitching, weakness, or facial numbness, dryness of the eye or the mouth, and/or disturbance of taste or hearing.

Clinical features

There is:
- unilateral paralysis of the upper and lower face (Figure 48.1)
- diminished blinking and absence of tearing
- sensation intact on testing.

Diagnosis

Bell palsy is a diagnosis by exclusion of other causes (Figure 48.2) (Table 48.1). Investigations should include:
- Neurological examination.
- Ear and mouth examination to exclude Ramsay Hunt's syndrome; herpes zoster of the facial nerve ganglion (geniculate ganglion), which causes lesions in the palate and ipsilateral ear, and facial palsy.
- Test for the degree of nerve damage; facial nerve stimulation or needle electromyography may be useful, as may electrogustometry, nerve excitability tests, electromyography and electroneuronography.
- Test for loss of hearing; pure tone audiometry is often used.
- Test for taste loss.
- Test for balance.
- Schirmer test for amount of tear production (lacrimation).
- MRI or CT imaging of the internal auditory meatus, cerebellopontine angle and mastoid.
- Chest radiography – to exclude sarcoidosis.

- Blood pressure measurement.
- Blood tests: Fasting blood sugar levels tests to exclude diabetes; serology to exclude HSV or other virus infections such as HIV; serum angiotensin converting enzyme (SACE) levels to exclude sarcoidosis; serum antinuclear antibodies (ANA) to exclude connective tissue disease; and enzyme-linked immunosorbent assay (ELISA) for *B. burgdorferi*.
- Occasionally, a lumbar puncture is required to exclude meningitis.

Management

Medical: Most patients improve spontaneously, but the effects in the remaining 15% can be so severe that active treatment is warranted. Systemic corticosteroids produce complete recovery in 80–90%. Antivirals (usually acyclovir or famciclovir) have also been advocated, but a large randomized trial in 2007 reported no additional benefit from aciclovir beyond that from corticosteroids. An eye pad should be worn to prevent corneal damage due to inadequate eyelid closure.

Trigeminal sensory loss

Facial and/or oral sensory loss is caused by lesions affecting the trigeminal nerve or central connections (Box 48.1), making the patient liable to self-injury.

The most common causes are extracranial and include damage following trauma (e.g. assaults, accidents, orthognathic, cancer or third molar surgery); disease in bone (osteomyelitis, malignant disease, Paget disease); drugs; diabetes; and multiple sclerosis.

Intracranial causes are uncommon but serious, and include trauma (including surgical treatment of trigeminal neuralgia); inflammatory disorders (sarcoidosis, infections such as HIV or syphilis, connective tissue disorders); malignant disease; cerebrovascular disease; drugs; diabetes; syringobulbia; multiple sclerosis and benign trigeminal neuropathy (etiology unknown, though some patients prove to have connective tissue disorder) and psychogenic causes.

Trigeminal pathology may cause ipsilateral pain as well as sensory loss, in the trigeminal trophic syndrome (TTS) caused mainly by trigeminal neuralgia surgery, lateral medullary infarction (Wallenberg syndrome) or zoster. Gabapentin may be effective therapy. Unilateral chin numbness (Numb chin syndrome (NCS)) may be caused by malignant infiltration of the inferior alveolar nerve by jaw metastases or local tumor (mainly lymphomas or breast cancer); infection such as osteomyelitis; a metastatic deposit at the level of the base of skull involving the mandibular division of the trigeminal nerve; metastasis to the meninges or as part of a paraneoplastic syndrome (Figure 48.3). Bilateral chin numbness, or circumoral numbness may be caused by hyperventilation, hypocalcemia or syringobulbia.

Imaging is invariably indicated; DPT, and CT or MRI of the brain and skull base and mandibular division of the trigeminal nerve, or scintiscanning may be appropriate. If imaging fails, lumbar puncture to exclude carcinomatous meningitis or leptomeningeal metastases may be necessary. Blood tests may be needed to exclude connective tissue disease or other causes.

49

Neurological conditions and pain: Local, referred and vascular

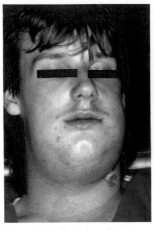

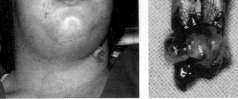

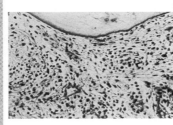

Abscess histology.

Figure 49.1a Facial swelling in acute periapical abscess.

Figure 49.1b Periapical abscess.

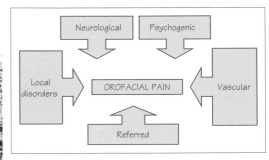

Figure 49.2 Causes of orofacial pain.

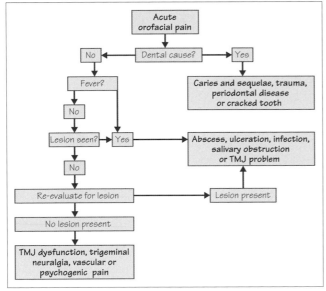

Figure 49.3a Acute pain diagnosis.

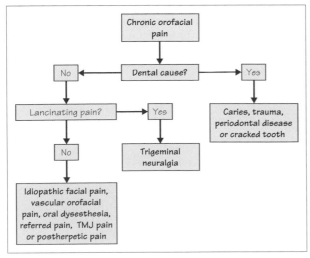

Figure 49.3b Chronic pain diagnosis.

Pain can vary in type (e.g. throbbing, burning, dull, stabbing), episodicity, and severity or intensity. The International Headache Society (IHS) defines pain intensity on a verbal scale (Table 49.1).

Orofacial pain is mediated by afferent fibers in trigeminal, nervus intermedius, glossopharyngeal, vagus and upper cervical nerves and may thus arise from pathology in their distributions. Orofacial pain is common, and mostly has obvious local causes (Figures 49.1a and b) but others are summarized in Figure 49.2.

Diagnosis

The diagnosis of orofacial pain is usually from the history and pain features (Figures 49.3a and b).

For example, odontogenic pain may be throbbing with an obvious location, trigeminal neuralgia is lancinating (stabbing) and unilateral, but idiopathic facial pain tends to be dull and may be bilateral (Chapter 51; Table 49.2).

Examination findings and imaging using radiography, CT, MRI or ultrasonography are important to avoid missing detecting organic disease and thus mislabeling the patient as having psychogenic pain. Even patients with psychogenic disorders can suffer organic pain: "Hypochondriacs can be ill"!

Medical advice should be urgently sought if orofacial pain is:
- accompanied by pain elsewhere (chest, shoulder, neck or arm – may be angina)
- accompanied by other unexplained symptoms or signs (numbness, weakness, headaches, neck stiffness, nausea or vomiting – may be intracerebral disease)
- focused in the temple on one side (may be giant cell arteritis).

Management

It is important to identify and treat the underlying cause of the pain. There is considerable individual variation in response to pain, and the threshold is lowered by tiredness, psychogenic and other factors, but treatment is generally helped by reassurance and:
- paracetamol, NSAIDs or other simple analgesics if the pain has an odontogenic cause
- triptans or other medications if pain is of vascular origin
- anticonvulsants if pain is neuralgic
- antidepressants if pain is of psychogenic origin.

Local causes of orofacial pain

Dental textbooks cover this important area (Table 49.3).

Table 49.1 IHS pain scores.

Scale	Pain	Consequences
0	None	None
1	Mild	Does not interfere with usual activities
2	Moderate	Inhibits, but does not wholly prevent usual activities
3	Severe	Prevents all usual activities

Table 49.2 Features of pain of different causes.

Pain is often	
Episodic	**Constant**
Odontogenic dentinal pain	Odontogenic pulpal pain
Trigeminal neuralgias	Idiopathic facial pain
Herpetic neuralgia	Burning mouth syndrome
Vascular pain	Temporomandibular pain-dysfunction
Referred anginal pain	

Referred causes of orofacial pain

Pain may occasionally be referred from the:
- Eyes: For example, refraction disorders, retrobulbar neuritis (multiple sclerosis), or glaucoma (raised intraocular pressure).
- Ears: For example, middle-ear disease.
- Styloid process (stylalgia): For example, Eagle syndrome, a rare disorder due to an elongated styloid process, causing pain on chewing, swallowing or turning the head.
- Neck: For example, cervical vertebral disease.
- Pharynx: For example, carcinoma of the pharynx.
- Lungs: For example, lung cancer.
- Heart: For example, angina.
- Esophagus: For example, esophagitis.

Vascular causes of orofacial pain (Table 49.4)

Both vascular and neural influences cause migraines and migrainous neuralgia. Stress triggers brain changes, serotonin (5-hydroxytryptamine) is released, blood vessels constrict and chemicals, including substance P, cause pain.

Giant cell arteritis is an inflammatory condition that affects arteries, in particular the temporal and optic artery, thus can lead to a sudden loss of vision. It usually only affects people over the age of 55 and is most common in people over 75, particularly women. Often people with polymyalgia rheumatica develop giant cell arteritis, but it can often occur on its own. The first sign may be pain on chewing, or headache usually concentrated in the temple – which may be tender to touch. Diagnosis is supported by raised ESR, and arteritis on biopsy. It is a medical concern needing corticosteroid treatment.

Table 49.3 Differential diagnosis of oral pain.

Source of pain	Character	Exacerbating factors	Ability to locate signs	Associated with	Pain provoked by	Imaging
Dental						
Dentinal	Evoked, does not outlast	Hot/cold Sweet or sour	Poor	Caries, defective restorations Exposed dentine	Hot/cold Probing dentine	May show interproximal caries Defective restorations
Pulpal	Severe, intermittent, throbbing	Hot/cold Sometimes biting	Poor	Deep caries Extensive restoration	Hot/cold, probing Sometimes percussion	May show deep caries or deep restoration
Periodontal						
Periapical	For hours at same intensity, deep, boring	Biting	Good	Periapical swelling and redness, tooth mobility	Percussion palpation of periapical area	Periapical views may show periapical changes
Lateral	For hours at same level Boring	Biting	Good	Periodontal swelling Deep pockets with pus exuding Tooth mobility	Percussion palpation of periodontal area	Useful when X-rayed with probe inserted into pocket
Gingival	Pressing Annoying	Food impaction Toothbrushing	Good	Acute gingival inflammation	Touch Percussion	Not applicable
Mucosal						
Mucosal	Burning, sharp	Sour, sharp and hot food	Good	Erosive or ulcerative lesions Redness	Palpation	Not applicable

Table 49.4 Important types of vascular orofacial pain.

	Migraine	Migrainous neuralgia	Giant cell arteritis
Other terms		Sluder, or cluster headaches	Horton disease, cranial or temporal arteritis
Age (years)	Any	30–50	> 50
Gender	F > M	M > F	F > M
Main pain location	Head and face, especially supraorbital	Retro-orbital	Temple
Pain character	Throbbing	Boring	Burning Tender, swollen arteries
Pain intensity	Severe	Severe	Severe
Pain duration	Hours (usually daytime)	Few hours (usually night)	Hours
Associated features	± Photophobia ± nausea ± vomiting Increased risk of stroke	Conjunctival injection ± lacrimation ± nasal congestion	± Visual loss Polymyalgia rheumatica
Investigations indicated	—	—	ESR and interleukin-6 raised Artery biopsy Ultrasound MRI
Precipitating factors	± Foods ± Stress	± Alcohol	—
Relieving factors	Sumatriptan Clonidine Ergot alkaloids	Oxygen Sumatriptan Clonidine Ergot alkaloids Verapamil	Corticosteroids (do not await investigation results before starting)

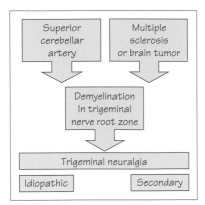

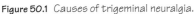

Figure 50.1 Causes of trigeminal neuralgia.

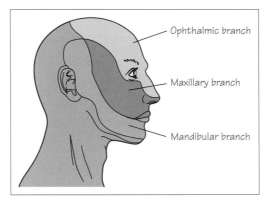

Figure 50.2a Trigeminal dermatomes.

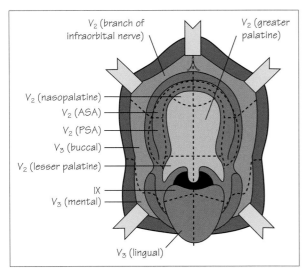

Figure 50.2b Intraoral innervations. ASA, anterior superior alveolar; PSA, posterior superior alveolar.

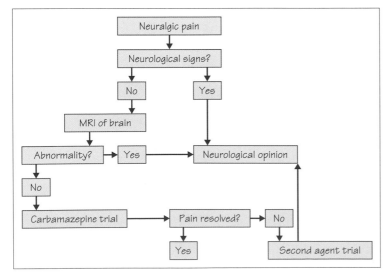

Figure 50.3 Management of neuralgia.

Pain of a neurological origin in the trigeminal area is termed trigeminal neuralgia (TN). The cause may be clear, when it is termed secondary TN, but usually no cause is evident; it is then idiopathic (ITN) or simply TN (Figure 50.1).

Trigeminal neuralgia

This includes idiopathic or benign paroxysmal trigeminal neuralgia, tic douloureux, prosopalgia.

Definition: Recurrent attacks of lancinating pain in the distribution of a trigeminal nerve division.

Prevalence (approximate): 1 per 15,000.

Age mainly affected: 50–70 year age group.

Gender mainly affected: F > M.

Etiopathogenesis: Trigeminal neuralgia (TN) appears to result from demyelination causing abnormal nerve signal transmission. In 90–95% of cases, no neurological lesion is identified, and the condition is then labeled ITN. The cause of ITN may be the superior cerebellar artery becoming atherosclerotic and less flexible, pressing on the trigeminal nerve roots in the posterior cranial fossa, damaging the myelin sheath. Demyelination may also be caused by multiple sclerosis (MS), cerebrovascular disease with pontine or medullary infarcts, neoplasms, aneurysms, cysts, trauma, infections, deposits such as amyloidosis or other causes (secondary TN). Some 2% of patients with MS develop TN. Hypertension is increased in patients with TN.

Clinical features

International Headache Society (IHS) defines the characteristics of TN as paroxysmal attacks of pain which last a few seconds to < 2 minutes, especially in the morning, rarely at night. Typical TN pain has the following features:

- intermittent
- unilateral
- distribution along one or more trigeminal division (Figures 50.2a and b)
- a sudden intense, sharp superficial, stabbing or burning quality
- severe intensity
- precipitation from trigger areas or daily activities affecting the trigeminal area such as eating, talking, washing the face, shaving or cleaning the teeth.

TN follows the sensory distribution of the trigeminal, usually radiating to the maxillary (V2), sometimes the mandibular (V3) and rarely to the ophthalmic (V1) division. Most patients develop the pain in one division, but over years the pain may travel through the other divisions; 10–12% of cases are bilateral, or occur on both sides. The attacks are stereotyped in the individual patient, tend to occur in cycles, with remissions lasting months or even years, but typically worsen in frequency or severity over time. Emotional or physical stress can increase the frequency and severity of TN attacks. The patient is usually entirely asymptomatic between paroxysms, though some do experience a dull ache.

A less common form, called "atypical TN", occasionally precedes the onset of mixed connective tissue disease (MCTD). It causes less intense, constant, dull burning or aching pain, sometimes with occasional electric-shock-like stabs, usually unilaterally, but sometimes bilaterally.

Diagnosis

Post-herpetic neuralgia, glossopharyngeal neuralgia, idiopathic facial pain, and dental problems, should particularly be excluded. Secondary TN from MS, cerebrovascular disease, space-occupying lesions such as neoplasms or aneurysms, or viral infections such as HIV or Lyme disease must be excluded, but then there may be physical signs such as facial sensory or motor impairment or loss of the corneal reflex. The following are indicated (Figure 50.3):

- History.
- Examination, including neurological assessment, especially of the cranial nerves.
- Investigations, including:
  — Imaging: Most physicians recommend elective MRI (gives better resolution of brain stem and cranial nerves than CT) of the entire trigeminal nerve for all patients and it is certainly mandatory if atypical features are present.
  — Blood tests: Erythrocyte sedimentation rate (ESR) to exclude vasculitides, anti-RNP antibodies for MCTD, and serology for Lyme disease or, rarely, HIV.

Only if all imaging and blood investigations prove negative can a diagnosis of ITN be made.

Management

Few patients have spontaneous remission; thus treatment is usually indicated and there is evidence that suggests the need to treat quickly. Anticonvulsants, especially carbamazepine, are successful for most ITN. Carbamazepine effectiveness may almost be regarded as diagnostic, but it must be given continuously prophylactically with monitoring for adverse effects (ataxia, drowsiness, gastrointestinal effects, folate deficiency, hyponatremia, hypertension, rashes, pancytopenia or rarely leukopenia) to control the dose. Carbamazepine should be avoided in Han Chinese (who may also react to phenytoin, and lamotrigine), because of a strong association between HLA-B*1502 allele and carbamazepine-induced Stevens-Johnson syndrome.

Some use baclofen as it has fewer adverse effects, and the combination with carbamazepine may provide relief. If these therapies fail, there are many effective alternatives or additions (clonazepam, gabapentin, lamotrigine, oxcarbazepine, phenytoin, pimozide, pregabaline, valproic acid). Surgical options include:

- *Peripheral nerve surgery* (cryosurgery, radiofrequency thermocoagulation or injections of glycerol or alcohol) may bring temporary relief.
- *Percutaneous approaches* inserting a needle through the face into the skull for trigeminal gangliolysis carry less risk and cost but pain is exchanged for anesthesia (risk of damage to the cornea) and, sometimes, anesthesia with pain (anesthesia dolorosa). Radiofrequency lesioning (RFL, percutaneous radiofrequency trigeminal gangliolysis (PRTG)), Fogarty balloon microcompression (FBM), and retrogasserian glycerol rhizotomy (PRGR) are percutaneous choices. Gamma knife stereotactic radiosurgery, however, is the least invasive procedure, with a high rate of pain control and fewest adverse effects, though potential disadvantages include its use of radiation and the fact that benefit often takes six weeks or more for success.
- *Open surgical procedures* include posterior cranial fossa procedures (microvascular decompression of the trigeminal root (MVD) and retrogasserian rhizotomy) – effective and with less chance of anesthesia, but with possible morbidity and even mortality.

51

Neurological conditions and pain: Psychogenic (idiopathic facial pain, idiopathic odontalgia, and burning mouth syndrome (oral dysesthesia))

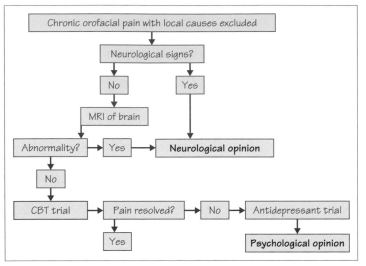

Chronic orofacial pain with local causes excluded

Neurological signs?

No → Yes

MRI of brain

Abnormality? → Yes → Neurological opinion

No

CBT trial → Pain resolved? → No → Antidepressant trial

Yes

Psychological opinion

Figure 51.1 Management of idiopathic facial pain (IFP). CBT, cognitive behavioural therapy.

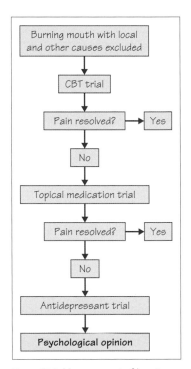

Figure 51.2 Pernicious anemia glossitis causing burning sensation.

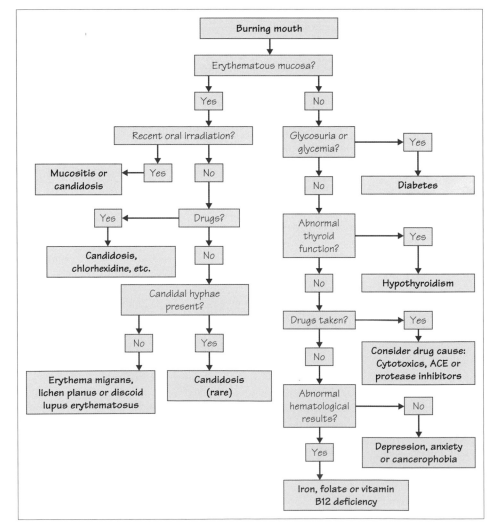

Burning mouth

Erythematous mucosa?

Yes → No

Recent oral irradiation?

Glycosuria or glycemia? → Yes

Mucositis or candidosis ← Yes → No

No → Diabetes

Yes ← Drugs? → No

Abnormal thyroid function? → Yes

Candidosis, chlorhexidine, etc.

No

No → Hypothyroidism

Candidal hyphae present?

Drugs taken? → Yes

No → Yes

No

Erythema migrans, lichen planus or discoid lupus erythematosus

Candidosis (rare)

Consider drug cause: Cytotoxics, ACE or protease inhibitors

Abnormal hematological results? → No

Yes

Depression, anxiety or cancerophobia

Iron, folate or vitamin B12 deficiency

Burning mouth with local and other causes excluded

CBT trial

Pain resolved? → Yes

No

Topical medication trial

Pain resolved? → Yes

No

Antidepressant trial

Psychological opinion

Figure 51.4 Management of burning mouth syndrome.

Figure 51.3 Diagnosis in burning mouth. ACE, angiotensin converting enzyme.

Persistent idiopathic, or unexplained (atypical) facial pain (IFP)

Definition: A constant chronic (> 6 months) orofacial discomfort or pain, defined by the IHS (International Headache Society) as "facial pain not fulfilling other criteria".

Prevalence (approximate): 0.5–1% of population.

Age mainly affected: Middle-age or older.

Gender mainly affected: F > M.

Etiopathogenesis: IFP falls into the category of medically unexplained symptoms (MUS). Most MUS seem to have no known organic cause, rather a psychogenic basis, but a patient suffering pain may well also manifest psychological reactions to it. Most sufferers are or have been under extreme stress, such as concern about cancer, a few have hypochondriases, neuroses (often depression) or psychoses.

Positron emission tomography shows increased brain activity, suggesting an enhanced alerting which may lead to neuropeptide release and free radical production, which might cause cell damage and release of pain-inducing eicosanoids (e.g. prostaglandins).

Diagnostic features

History

Oral: IFP is often a dull boring or burning continuous poorly localised pain (rarely as severe as trigeminal neuralgia). The pain persists during the day, but does not disturb sleep. The pain is confined initially to a limited area (unrelated to the trigeminal nerve distribution) on one side only, but may spread. Other characteristics are a lack of objective signs, and a poor treatment response. There are often also multiple oral complaints, such as dry mouth and bad taste.

Idiopathic, or atypical odontalgia (IO), a prolonged or throbbing pain in the teeth or alveolar process in the absence of any identifiable odontogenic cause, has been considered a variety of IFP.

Extraoral: Often also headaches, chronic back pain, irritable bowel syndrome and/or dysmenorrhea. There is a high level of utilization of health care services with multiple consultations and treatment attempts.

Clinical features

Oral: None.

Extraoral: None.

Differential diagnosis: Other causes of orofacial pain.

Careful dental, otolaryngological, and neurological examination, and imaging (tooth/jaw/sinus/skull radiography and MRI/CT scan of the head with particular attention to skull base) to exclude space-occupying or demyelinating diseases are indicated.

Only if all imaging studies prove negative can a diagnosis of IFP be made.

Management

Few patients have spontaneous remission and thus treatment is indicated. The clinician should never trivialize or dismiss the patient's symptoms. Cognitive-behavioural therapy (CBT) or a specialist referral may be indicated (Figure 51.1). "Reattribution" helps; this involves demonstrating an understanding of the complaints, making the patient feel understood and supported, and widening the agenda, thereby making the link between symptoms and psychological problems. It may help to explain that depression/tiredness lower pain thresholds and that muscle spasm ("being uptight") produces pain. It is best to avoid repeat examinations or investigations which only serve to reinforce illness behavior and health fears. A trial of an antidepressant such as dosulepine, amitriptyline or moclobemide may be warranted, explaining that these are used to treat the pain rather than any depression. Acupuncture and transcutaneous electrical nerve stimulation (TENS) have been also recommended.

Prognosis
Variable.

Burning mouth "syndrome" (BMS, glossopyrosis, glossodynia, oral dysesthesia, scalded mouth syndrome, or stomatodynia)

Definition: A burning mouth sensation may be a primary condition, or secondary to identifiable causes (Figure 51.2). Burning mouth syndrome (BMS) is the term used when symptoms exist in the absence of identifiable organic etiological factors; it is a MUS. The IHS define it as "an intraoral burning sensation for which no medical or dental cause can be found".

Prevalence (approximate): 5 persons per 100,000.

Age mainly affected: Middle age or older.

Gender mainly affected: F > M.

Etiopathogenesis: No precipitating cause for BMS can be identified in over 50% of patients and it has been suggested that it is related to nerve damage or reduced pain thresholds. A psychogenic cause, such as anxiety, depression or cancerophobia, can be identified in about 20%. BMS is increased in frequency in Parkinsonism and, in some, it appears to follow dental intervention, respiratory infection, or exposure to various substances or drugs (e.g. angiotensin converting enzyme (ACE) inhibitors or protease inhibitors (PIs)).

Diagnostic features

History

Oral: BMS most frequently affects the tongue but it can also affect the palate, lips or lower alveolus. The complaint is usually persistent and bilateral and worsens as the day progresses, but does not disturb sleep. It is often relieved by eating and drinking, in contrast to pain caused by organic lesions (aggravated by eating). BMS may ameliorate during working or with distractions. There are often also multiple psychogenic-related complaints, such as dry mouth and bad or altered taste (bitter or metallic).

Extraoral: May also be headaches, chronic back pain, irritable bowel syndrome, dysmenorrhea and changes in sleep patterns and mood, and there have often already been multiple consultations and treatment attempts ("doctor-shopping").

Clinical features

Oral: None.

Extraoral: None.

Differential diagnosis: Conditions that can also present with burning should be excluded (Figure 51.3). IHS diagnostic criteria for BMS are:

* pain in the mouth present daily and persisting for most of the day
* oral mucosa is of normal appearance
* local and systemic diseases have been excluded

Only if all investigations prove negative can BMS be diagnosed.

Management

About 50% of patients with BMS remit spontaneously within about six years, but few have spontaneous remission in the short term; thus treatment is usually indicated (Figure 51.4). Management is as for IFP but some patients respond to CBT, or to topical benzydamine rinse or spray, capsaicin cream, or a sucked clonazepam tablet. Antidepressants may be needed.

Prognosis
Variable.

52

Jaw conditions: Temporomandibular pain-dysfunction

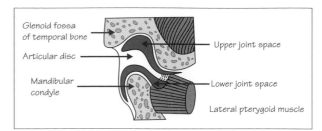

Figure 52.1a TMJ anatomy.

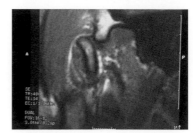

Figure 52.1b Temporomandibular joint.

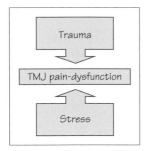

Figure 52.2 Causes of TMJ dysfunction.

Table 52.1 Main causes of restricted jaw opening.

Extra-articular	Intra-articular
Condylar neck fracture	Ankylosis
Coronoid hypertrophy	Condylar intracapsular fracture
Fibrosis (scar, scleroderma, submucous fibrosis)	Joint arthritis, dislocation or subluxation
Hysteria	
Masticatory muscle infection, hematoma or inflammation	
Neoplasm	
Temporomandibular joint dysfunction	
Tetanus	
Tetany	

Table 52.2 Investigations used in temporomandibular joint disease.

Procedure	Advantages	Disadvantages
Arthrography (double contrast)	Provides excellent information	Danger of infection Painful
Arthroscopy	Good visualization Minimally invasive	Requires anesthesia Technically demanding
Magnetic resonance imaging (MRI)	Excellent information without exposure to ionising radiation Non-invasive	Expensive Not universally available
Radiography	Simple, can reveal much pathology DPT demonstrates both TMJs CT, especially cone beam, can provide excellent information	— Expensive
Ultrasonography	Non-invasive	Role doubtful

The temporomandibular joint (TMJ) has a complex anatomy (Figures 52.1a and b). Limited opening of the jaw (sometimes termed trismus) may have several causes (Table 52.1).

Investigations available to help diagnose TMJ disorders are shown in Table 52.2.

Temporomandibular joint pain-dysfunction syndrome (TMPD), myofascial pain dysfunction (MFD), facial arthromyalgia (FAM), mandibular dysfunction, or mandibular stress syndrome

TMPD is one of the most common complaints but also one of the most controversial areas in dentistry.

Definition: Refers to a common triad of temporomandibular joint (TMJ) symptoms – clicking, jaw locking (or limitation of opening) and pain.

Prevalence (approximate): Up to 12% of the population.

Age mainly affected: Teens and up to 20–40 years of age.

Gender mainly affected: F > M.

Etiopathogenesis: Trauma and stress appear to predispose through increasing tension affecting the masticatory muscles (Figure 52.2). Acute trauma can occasionally precede TMJ dysfunction but more commonly, prolonged and/or excessive mandibular opening, habits such as chewing a pen, or parafunctions (e.g. day-time jaw clenching or night-time tooth grinding (bruxism)) lead to it. Depression and shortage of sleep are considered important risk indicators.

Abnormalities in dental occlusion are controversial as causes as there is no neurophysiological evidence to support a primary etiological role for the occlusion and many people with gross malocclusions have no TMJ dysfunction, nor is there any evidence for a relationship between orthodontic treatment (or the wearing of orthodontic headgear) and TMJ dysfunction.

Displacement of the TMJ meniscus (internal disc derangement (IDD)) is common, and can be demonstrated by MRI and arthroscopy but may be seen in asymptomatic TMJs. With mouth opening, the disc may be reduced (recaptured) or remain displaced.

Diagnostic features

History

Oral: Symptoms are highly variable, but the following are characteristic:
- *Recurrent joint clicking*: Either on opening or closing, but are not diagnostic, being common in normal joints.
- *Limitation of jaw movement*: May be intermittent, with jaw deviation to the affected side on attempted opening, or "locking".
- *Pain*: Typically unilateral, in the joint region, can radiate to the back of the mouth, neck, temple or behind the ear (areas of V3 sensory innervations).

Symptoms can be quantified by the Helkimo indices based on both patient information (anamnestic dysfunction index, Ai) and clinical findings (clinical dysfunction index, Di).

Extraoral; Some patients may also complain of headaches, neck aches, and lower back pain.

Clinical features

Oral: There may be crepitus from the TMJ, limited or deviated opening, clicking or popping in the TMJ and/or diffuse tenderness or spasm on palpation of masseter, temporalis, medial or lateral pterygoid muscles.

Differential diagnosis: Rheumatoid arthritis, osteoarthritis, or other TMJ pathology.

Diagnosis is mainly on clinical grounds. The occlusion and any dental appliances should be assessed. Imaging is rarely indicated, only where there is:
- a history of trauma
- significant limitation of movement
- sensory or motor alteration
- a real possibility of organic joint or other disease.

MRI is most useful if looking for disc pathology; CT may reveal greater bone detail. The condylar position is unreliable for diagnosis and does not indicate meniscus displacement. There is no reliable evidence to support use of other suggested diagnostic "aids".

Management

TMJ dysfunction appears not to lead to long-term joint damage, and many patients have spontaneous remission. Thus treatment is not always indicated but may be worthwhile in persons who have pain. Conservative measures are at least partially successful in up to 90%. Treatment aims to:
- control immediate pain with analgesics (very occasionally injections of local analgesics or corticosteroids may be required)
- reduce psychological stress (by reassurance)
- eliminate TMJ damage (by rest).

A typical conservative regimen includes use of:
- soft diet
- rest and avoidance of trauma, wide-opening and abnormal habits
- warmth, massage and remedial jaw exercises
- non-steroidal anti-inflammatory agents, e.g. aspirin.

If these are insufficient, it may be helpful to use:
- muscle relaxants
- hard plastic splints on the occlusal surfaces (occlusal splints).

The 5–10% of patients who fail to respond to this treatment may need treatment for psychological problems by either medication or psychiatric therapy.

Surgery may be required for the extremely small number of remaining non-responders, or those with obvious intra-articular pathology (e.g. osteoarthritis).

However, a huge range of other "treatment" options is offered for TMJ dysfunction, indicating that few are specific or reliably effective.

Prognosis

Some patients' symptoms may resolve within weeks; others have chronic symptoms; and about one-third of patients have recurrent episodes.

53

Jaw bone conditions: Radiolucencies and radiopacities

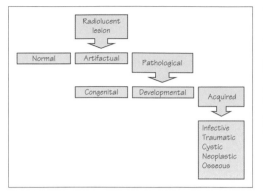

Figure 53.1a Radiolucent lesions.

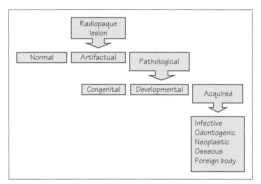

Figure 53.4a Radiopaque lesions.

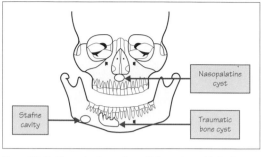

Figure 53.1b Nonodontogenic radiolucent cystic lesions.

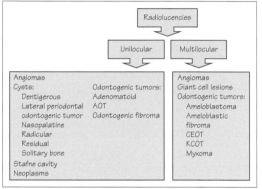

Figure 53.4b Radiolucent lesions. CEOT, calcifying epithelial odontogenic tumor; KCOT, keratocystic odontogenic tumor; AOT, adenomatoid odontogenic tumor.

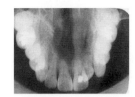

Figure 53.2 Nasopalatine duct cyst.

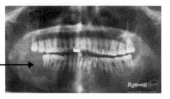

Figure 53.3 Hyperparathyroidism. Brown tumor.

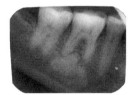

Figure 53.5 Osteosclerosis.

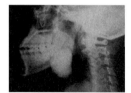

Figure 53.6a Osteoma.

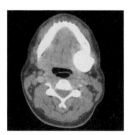

Figure 53.6b CT Osteoma.

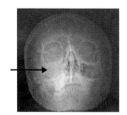

Figure 53.7 Osteosarcoma.

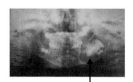

Figure 53.8 Ameloblastic fibro-odontoma.

Many diseases of or in the jaws present asymptomatically as *radiolucencies*, *radiopacities* or with mixed appearances on imaging. Other presentations are as *swellings*, *pain* or sometimes *fracture* or *disturbance of tooth eruption* (displaced, missing or loose teeth). Swellings that appear to originate from the jaws may arise from subcutaneous tissues or bones: the mnemonic MINT aids diagnosis:

Malformations, e.g. tori and fibro-osseous lesions
Inflammatory conditions, e.g. odontogenic infections, osteomyelitis, actinomycosis, tuberculosis, or syphilis
Neoplasms and cysts (see below)
Trauma causing subperiosteal hematomas

Investigations largely involve imaging, and serum calcium, phosphate, and alkaline phosphatase levels, but histopathology is almost invariably required (Tables 53.1 and 53.2).

Radiolucencies

Radiographic features to be assessed include the lesional size, shape, number, margins, character (radiolucency and/or radiopacity), and effects (displacement of the inferior alveolar nerve or tooth displacement or resorption).

Well-defined radiolucencies are often odontogenic cysts and benign tumors.

Poorly defined radiolucencies are often infections or tumors.

Jaw radiolucencies may include (Figures 53.1a and b):

• *Odontogenic diseases*, inflammation, cysts and tumors (Chapter 54).
• *Non-odontogenic cysts*, e.g. nasopalatine duct cyst (in maxillary midline, with a characteristic heart shape) (Figure 53.2), and traumatic bone cyst (solitary, simple, hemorrhagic bone cyst).
• *Vascular or neurogenic lesions*:
— *Arteriovenous malformation*: Abnormal communication between arteries and veins, or central hemangioma.
— *Central giant cell granuloma*: Initially a small, unilocular radiolucency, eventually becoming multilocular, and may then mimic

hyperparathyroidism brown tumors (Figure 53.3) (histologically similar). Biochemistry distinguishes these entities.

— *Neurofibroma*: May present as widening of inferior alveolar canal.
• *Metabolic disorders*: Osteoporosis, osteomalacia, renal osteodystrophy, osteitis fibrosa cystica (hyperparathyroidism).
• *Malignant tumors* include squamous cell carcinomas (invading mainly from mouth or antrum), osteosarcomas (a symmetrically widened periodontal membrane in a single tooth may be earliest indication), lymphomas (ill-defined lesions), and multiple myeloma ("punched-out" ovoid lesions).
• *Metastases* from kidney, lung, and breast tumors (but 30% originate from an occult primary lesion) typically have ill-defined borders.

Radiopacities

Radiopaque lesions include (Figures 53.4a and 4b):
• *Unerupted teeth.*
• *Foreign bodies.*
• *Congenital and developmental anomalies*, e.g., torus and other bone lumps. Gardner syndrome (colorectal polyposis, tumors, and skeletal abnormalities) is an autosomal dominant condition caused by APC gene mutation, with osteomas and often impacted and supernumerary teeth and odontomas. Carriers may have jaw radiopacities.
• *Odontogenic cysts and tumors* (Chapter 54 and 55).
• *Fibro-osseous lesions* (Chapter 57).
• *Inflamed and infected lesions*:
— Odontogenic infections
— *Osteomyelitis*: Shows no imaging findings until the acute inflammatory reaction leads to bone lysis (osteolysis). Bone density has to fall by 30–50% to show on plain radiography and this usually takes 2–3 weeks. Plain radiographs, and more accurately CT (either MDCT (multidetector CT) or CBCT (Cone Beam)) can demonstrate the osteopenia and cortical lysis (including the inferior alveolar canal and mental foramen), sequestra and periosteal new bone formation. MRI has high sensitivity in detecting cancellous marrow abnormalities. In osteomyelitis, periosteal new bone apposition causes cortical thickening and mandibular enlargement, most common on the buccal plate of the mandibular angle or body, especially in young people. Swelling of masseter and medial pterygoid muscles is common and both CT and MRI show soft-tissue inflammation especially in the masticatory and submandibular spaces. Bone scintigraphy (bone scan) is highly sensitive in detecting acute osteomyelitis but requires anatomical correlation. Technetium-labeled compounds depict bone turnover and radiolabeled leukocyte scans can confirm this is infection.
■ *Primary chronic osteomyelitis* shows extensive and diffuse sclerosis sometimes with expansion.
■ *Secondary chronic osteomyelitis* shows a mixed radiolucent and radiopaque appearance.

■ *Focal sclerosing osteomyelitis* (condensing osteitis).
■ *Chronic diffuse sclerosing osteomyelitis.*
— *Idiopathic osteosclerosis* (dense bone island): An area of dense bone in the jaw without apparent cause or signs or symptoms, typically seen in the mandibular premolar/molar area, may be associated with root resorption or Gardner syndrome (Figure 53.5).
— *Osteonecrosis*: This may follow radiation (osteoradionecrosis, ORN) or drug use (bisphosphonate-related osteochemonecrosis of the jaws, BRONJ).
— *Primary nonodontogenic tumors*: For example, osteomas (Figures 53.6a and b), and prostatic carcinoma metastases are often radiopaque. Sarcomas can cause osteolytic or osteoblastic lesions (Figure 53.7).

Mixed radiolucent and radiopaque lesions

Mixed radiolucent and radiopaque lesions are mainly fibro-osseous lesions, inflammatory processes (e.g. osteomyelitis, actinomycosis, osteonecrosis) and, less commonly, odontogenic tumors (Figure 53.8) (mainly adenomatoid odontogenic tumor and calcifying epithelial odontogenic tumor).

Table 53.2 Radiographic views for demonstrating various orofacial sites.

Region required	Standard views	Additional views
Facial bones	Occipital mental Occipital mental 30 Lateral	Zygoma Reduced exposure Submento vertex Lateral obliques
Mandible	Dental panoramic tomogram	PA mandible Mandibular occlusal
Maxilla	Occipital mental for maxillary antra	Upper occlusal or lateral Submento vertex DPT, tomography
Nasal bones	Occipital mental 30 Lateral Soft tissue lateral	
Skull	Posterior anterior 20 Lateral Townes (1/2 axial view)	Submento vertex Tangential
Temporomandibular joints	Transcranial lateral obliques or Dental panoramic tomogram (mouth open and closed)	Transpharyngeal Arthrography Reverse Townes Reverse DPT Consider MRI/CT scan/cone beam CT

Table 53.1 Investigations used in diseases of jaws.

Procedure	Advantages	Disadvantages	Remarks
Aspiration	Simple, using 18 gauge needle	May introduce infection	Cyst protein levels < 4 g% in KCOT
Bone biopsy	Definitive	Invasive	—
Bone scan	Surveys all skeleton	Those of any isotope procedure	May reveal metastases or osteomyelitis
Endoscopy (fibre-optic)	Simple, good visualization	Skill needed	Examines nasal passages, sinuses, pharynx and larynx
Imaging	Often simple	Can be expensive	

54

Jaw bone conditions: Odontogenic diseases and cysts

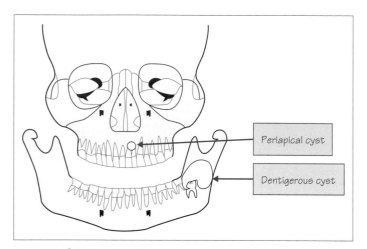

Figure 54.1 Odontogenic cysts.

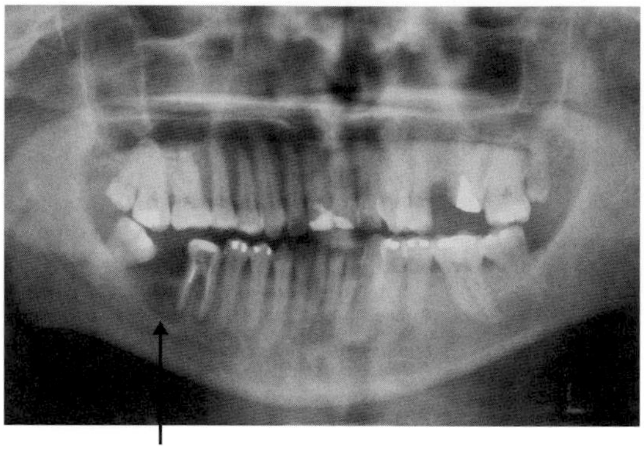

Periapical cyst

Dentigerous cyst

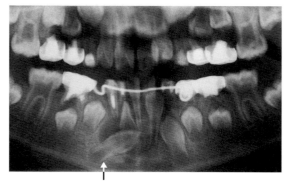

Figure 54.2a Apical cyst and granuloma.

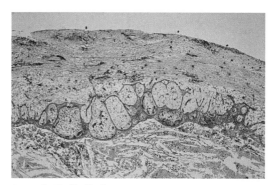

Figure 54.2b Radicular cyst.

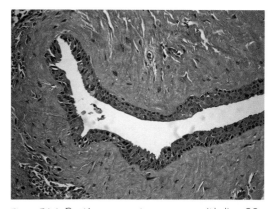

Figure 54.3 Dentigerous cyst.

Figure 54.4 Dentigerous cyst squamous epithelium 20 ×.

Table 54.1 Main odontogenic cysts.

Type	Decade at presentation	Commonest location	Usual management
Dentigerous	2nd to 4th	Lower third molars, maxillary canines	Enucleation or marsupialization
Eruption	1st	Anterior to permanent molars	Nil unless impeding eruption
Radicular	3rd & 4th	Anterior maxilla	Enucleation
Residual	4th & 5th	Anterior maxilla	Enucleation or marsupialization

Box 54.1 Jaw cysts.

Odontogenic Inflammatory	Developmental	Nonodontogenic	Pseudocysts
Buccal bifurcation cyst	Dentigerous cyst	Nasopalatine cyst	Hematopoietic bone marrow defect
Periapical granuloma and cyst	Eruption cyst		Static bone cyst
Residual cyst	Glandular odontogenic cyst		Traumatic bone cyst
	Lateral periodontal cyst		

Modified from Regezi JA (2002). Odontogenic cysts, odontogenic tumors, fibroosseous, and giant cell lesions of the jaws. *Mod Pathol,* **15** (3), 331–341.

Odontogenic diseases may be related to the tooth or its germ.

Odontogenic infections

Caries, periodontitis or pericoronitis are the common oral pyogenic infections. Depending on bacterial load and host immunity, dental pulpal infection may lead to apical periodontitis, abscess, and fascial space infection, or granuloma or periapical (radicular) cyst.

Odontogenic cysts

Odontogenic cysts (and tumors) arise from odontogenic ectoderm, mesenchyme or a combination (ectomesenchyme) and they may be at the site of a tooth germ, or associated with a tooth. There is a male predominance and the mandible is affected three times as commonly as the maxilla.

Clinical features: Often asymptomatic, cysts are usually an incidental finding on imaging, are generally benign, slow-growing and may reach large sizes before they give rise to:

• Swelling, initially a smooth bony hard lump with normal mucosa but, as bone thins, it may crackle on palpation like an egg shell. The cyst may resorb bone and show as a bluish fluctuant swelling.
• Discharge.
• Pain, if infected or if the jaw fractures pathologically.

Rarely, carcinomas may arise within some cysts.

Diagnosis: Most cysts are discovered on radiography. In the mandible they, by definition, arise above the inferior alveolar canal. MDCT, CBCT or MRI can help distinguish solid and cystic lesions. Other investigations may include pulp vitality testing, aspiration and analysis of cyst fluids, and histopathology.

Management: Enucleation (complete removal of the cyst) makes all tissue available for histological examination, the cavity usually heals uneventfully with minimal aftercare, but it may render adjacent teeth non-vital. Marsupialization (partial removal) requires considerable aftercare and patient cooperation in keeping the cavity clean – syringing after meals. Healing may take up to six months and not all cyst lining is available for histopathology (Table 54.1).

Odontogenic cysts are relatively common – most are inflammatory (55% of all) or dentigerous (22%) (Box 54.1) (Figure 54.1). Odontogenic cysts that can be problematical because of recurrence and/or aggressive growth include especially the glandular odontogenic cyst.

Periapical (radicular or dental) cyst is inflammatory, and the most common odontogenic cyst. It results from pulpal infections leading to periapical infection, a granuloma, and, finally, a cyst (Figures 54.2a and b). The epithelial lining is derived from the rests of Malassez and is thick, irregular, squamous epithelium, with granulation tissue forming the wall in denuded areas. There may be areas of chronic or acute inflammation with abscess formation. Cholesterol crystal clefts and mucous cells may be found. The cyst fluid is usually watery but may be thick and viscid with cholesterol crystal clefts. The cysts have capsules of fibrous connective tissue.

Characterized by its position at the apex of a non-vital tooth (pulp necrotic because of caries, trauma or deep restoration), there is a round or pear-shaped, well-defined radiolucent lesion with sclerotic borders, larger (often > 20 mm) than a periapical granuloma, with a rounder contour, and more well-defined border. It often involves a maxillary incisor or canine.

Any cyst that remains after surgery is termed a *residual cyst* – most arise from periapical cysts.

Follicular (dentigerous) cyst is the most common developmental odontogenic cyst (Figure 54.3). It forms from the follicle of an unerupted tooth and therefore, the tooth crown projects into the well-demarcated cavity lined by flattened stratified epithelium (a pericoronal position may also be seen in keratocystic odontogenic tumor (KCOT) and other benign tumors) (Figure 54.4). Follicular cysts are unilocular, radiolucent, and may become extremely large (more so than the radicular cyst) but, in contrast to a malignant lesion, cortical bone is usually preserved. A hyperplastic follicle in contrast, is < 5 mm, and neither displaces the tooth nor causes cortical expansion. A 2–3 mm follicle can be considered normal.

Rarely, mucoepidermoid carcinoma, ameloblastoma or squamous carcinoma have arisen from the walls of a follicular cyst; hence cyst removal is recommended.

Eruption cysts are minor soft tissue forms of dentigerous cysts. They often burst spontaneously. In some cases, the teeth are prevented from eruption by fibrous tissue overlying them.

Lateral periodontal cyst is small, and lateral to a vital tooth root, often in mandibular canine and premolar regions (*botryoid odontogenic cyst* is similar except that it is polycystic).

Buccal bifurcation cyst is centred on the first or second mandibular molar, often presenting with delayed tooth eruption.

Glandular odontogenic cyst (GOC, sialo-odontogenic cyst) is rare but may superficially mimic a central mucoepidermoid carcinoma. Features include epithelial whorls, cuboidal eosinophilic cells, goblet cells, ciliated cells and mucous pools which, with expression of p53 and Ki67, may aid the diagnosis. GOC tend to be aggressive and may recur following curettage.

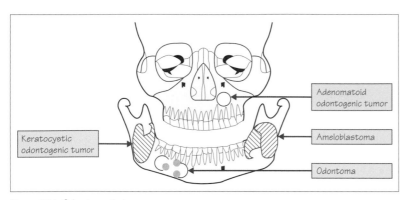

Figure 55.1 *Odontogenic tumors.*

Adenomatoid odontogenic tumor

Keratocystic odontogenic tumor

Ameloblastoma

Odontoma

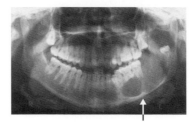

Figure 55.2 *Ameloblastoma (solid multicystic type).*

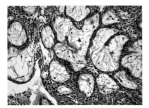

Figure 55.3 Plexiform ameloblastoma 20×.

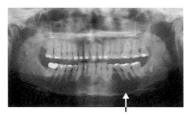

Figure 55.4 Keratocystic odontogenic tumor.

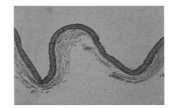

Figure 55.5 Keratocystic odontogenic tumor.

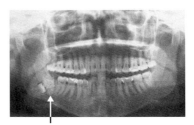

Figure 55.6a *Odontoma (odontome) complex.*

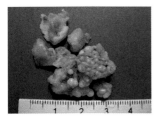

Figure 55.6b *Odontoma complex.*

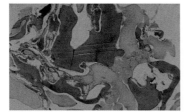

Figure 55.6c *Odontoma.*

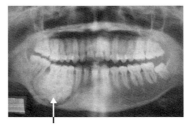

Figure 55.7 *Cementoblastoma.*

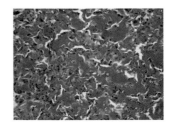

Figure 55.8 *Cementoblastoma.*

Odontogenic tumors are rare, are often asymptomatic, and discovered incidentally on imaging. They are generally slow-growing and may reach a large size before becoming symptomatic, for example:

• Swelling, sometimes with cortical perforation. Despite some odontogenic tumors expanding rather than destroying bone, there may be local invasion of surrounding bone.

• Pain, due to secondary infection or pathological fracture.

Management depends on the type of tumor, since odontogenic tumors may be either benign or malignant, and can be enucleation, dentoalveolar segmental resection with lower border of mandible preservation, segmental resection, or composite resection (Table 55.1).

Benign odontogenic tumors

Most frequent odontogenic tumors are keratocystic odontogenic tumors (Figure 55.1); most are odontomas (odontomes), or ameloblastomas.

Ameloblastoma predominates in the posterior mandible, presenting typically in third to fifth decades as a slow-growing, painless, uni- or multilocular mass ("soap-bubble" appearance on imaging) and producing more buccolingual expansion and root resorption than does keratocystic odontogenic tumor (but differentiation is difficult by radiography/CT) (Figure 55.2). MRI may then help. Ameloblastoma is regarded as benign but significant since it may recur or metastasize. Composed of ameloblast-like epithelial cells arranged as a peripheral layer around a central area resembling stellate reticulum, two main histological types exist. The *follicular* type contains discrete islands (follicles) of cells: the *plexiform* type consists of anastomosing strands (Figure 55.3). The treatment of choice is conservative resection with clear margins.

Squamous odontogenic tumor is rare and usually presents as a painless swelling and radiolucency between teeth which become mobile. It may mimic periodontal disease. Conservative excision is the treatment of choice.

Calcifying epithelial odontogenic tumor (CEOT, Pindborg tumor) is rare, benign but aggressive, though less than ameloblastoma. Distinct histological features include:

• sheets of pleomorphic epithelial cells, in places, characterized by clear cytoplasm ("clear cells")

• amyloid

• concentric masses of calcified tissues.

Usually seen in mandibular premolar or molar regions associated with the crown of an impacted tooth, CEOT is radiolucent with scattered calcified components. Conservative resection is the treatment of choice.

Adenomatoid odontogenic tumor is the "two-thirds tumor", most commonly noted in the second and third decades of life and two-thirds of cases:
- are in females
- occur in the anterior maxilla
- are associated with an impacted tooth (usually canine).

Sheets and strands of epithelial cells are arranged as convoluted bands and tubular structures, in which ameloblast-like cells are arranged radially around a homogeneous eosinophilic material. It presents as a well-demarcated unilocular radiolucent lesion often with punctate calcifications. The treatment of choice is enucleation and curettage, after which it rarely recurs.

Keratocystic odontogenic tumor (KCOT) is often unilocular but with a scalloped margin, well-defined, radiolucent, usually without an associated tooth (Figure 55.4) and benign, but with a propensity for local destruction and recurrence. The lining has a regular keratinised stratified squamous epithelium, five to eight cell layers thick and without rete pegs (Figure 55.5). Desquamated keratin is often present within the lumen and the fibrous wall is usually thin. The treatment of choice is surgery.

KCOT is associated with chromosome 9 PTCH gene mutations. Multiple KCOTs in young patients should suggest the basal cell nevus (Gorlin-Goltz) syndrome, an autosomal dominant disorder also with midface hypoplasia, frontal bossing and prognathism, falx cerebri calcification and skeletal anomalies.

Odontogenic myxoma is clinically and radiographically indistinguishable from ameloblastoma.

Ameloblastic fibroma consists of islands, elongated strands, or terminal buds of ameloblast-like cells and central stellate reticulum cells scattered in a mesenchyme-like cellular tissue. It is usually well-defined, pericoronal, multiloculated, radiolucent and associated with an impacted tooth, often in the posterior mandible.

Calcifying cystic odontogenic tumor (Gorlin cyst) is most common in the anterior jaw as a unilocular radiolucency. In one-third of cases, an impacted tooth is involved. Ghost cells – enlarged eosinophilic epithelial cells without nuclei – are a prominent feature. It may occasionally be aggressive/recurrent.

Odontoma (odontome), a "hamartoma" consisting of dentine and enamel, appears either in the maxilla or mandible, in the tooth bearing area, often associated with an impacted tooth. Odontomas are classified as:
- Compound type (compound composite odontomas) – multiple small simple denticles embedded in fibrous connective tissue within a capsule. Multiple lesions may be seen in Gardner syndrome.
- Complex type (complex composite odontomas) – an irregular mass of all dental tissues (Figures 55.6a–c).

Odontomas typically present during the second decade, and are more common in females than males. Typically, they can behave like teeth: they can grow and tend to erupt, or may displace adjacent teeth or impede their eruption. They are treated by local excision.

Cementoblastoma is a neoplasm of cementum typically seen in patients under 25 years. Usually fused to a root (typically mandibular premolar or first molar), it is a well-defined radiopacity with a radiolucent margin (Figures 55.7 and 55.8). It may cause pain which responds to NSAIDs. Hypercementosis in contrast, is smoother, less nodular, and has a thin radiolucent margin continuous with the periodontal ligament space.

Malignant odontogenic tumors

These are the malignant counterparts of the benign categories (Table 55.1).

Table 55.1 Odontogenic tumors.

Benign	Malignant
Odontogenic epithelium with mature, fibrous stroma without odontogenic ectomesenchyme	**Odontogenic carcinomas**
Ameloblastoma	Metastasizing (malignant) ameloblastoma
Squamous odontogenic tumor	Ameloblastic carcinoma
Calcifying epithelial odontogenic tumor	Primary intraosseous squamous cell carcinoma
Adenomatoid odontogenic tumor	Clear cell odontogenic carcinoma
Keratocystic odontogenic tumor (KCOT)	Ghost cell odontogenic carcinoma
Odontogenic epithelium with odontogenic ectomesenchyme, with or without hard tissue formation	**Odontogenic sarcomas**
Ameloblastic fibroma	Ameloblastic fibro sarcoma
Ameloblastic fibrodentinoma	Ameloblastic fibrodentino- and fibro-odontosarcoma
Ameloblastic fibro-odontoma	
Odontoma (odontome)	
Odontoameloblastoma	
Calcifying cystic odontogenic tumor	
Dentinogenic ghost cell tumor	
Mesenchyme and/or odontogenic ectomesenchyme with or without odontogenic epithelium	
Odontogenic fibroma	
Odontogenic myxoma/myxofibroma	
Cementoblastoma	

Adapted from World Health Organization (2005). Classification of odontogenic tumors. In: *International Statistical Classification of Diseases and Related Health Problems*. Geneva, WHO.

Jaw conditions: Bone disorders

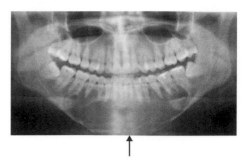

Figure 56.1a Solitary bone cyst.

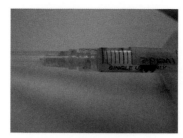

Figure 56.1b Solitary bone cyst aspirate.

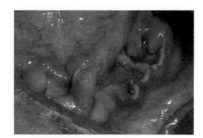

Figure 56.2 Bisphosphonate related osteonecrosis.

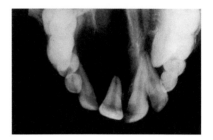

Figure 56.3a Giant cell granuloma.

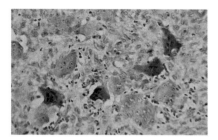

Figure 56.3b Giant cell granuloma.

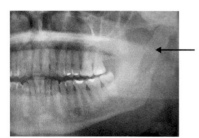

Figure 56.4 Langerhans cells histiocytosis lesions in ramus and condyle.

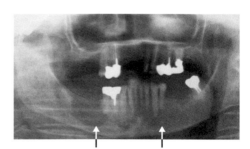

Figure 56.5a Multiple myeloma (from Bagan JV, Scully C. Medicina y Patologia Oral, 2006).

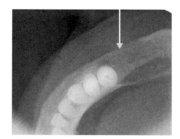

Figure 56.5b Multiple myeloma fracture of jaw through a lesion.

Table 56.1 Bone neoplasms.

Benign	Malignant
Chondroma	Chondrosarcoma
Osteoblastoma	Osteosarcoma
Osteochondroma	
Osteoma	

Some jaw bone conditions are "pseudo-diseases", such as unerupted teeth, bone marrow defects, Stafne bone defect (static bone cyst), osteosclerosis, pseudocyst of maxillary sinus, or sub-pontic osseous hyperplasia. Traumatic (solitary) bone cyst arises from trauma causing intramedullary hemorrhage that subsequently leaves a radiolucency with characteristic scalloped superior margin (it rarely damages teeth) (Figures 56.1a and b). Bone diseases that may affect the jaws are described below.

Non-neoplastic diseases

• *Osteonecrosis.* Osteoradionecrosis (ORN) and bisphosphonate-related osteochemonecrosis of the jaws (BRONJ) are uncommon complications of radiation therapy of head and neck tumors, and bisphosphonate use (especially when given intravenously) respectively. The bone repair response is impaired by these therapies, and surgical interventions (e.g. tooth extraction), may precipitate the osteonecrosis. Both manifest with exposed bone, loose teeth, discharge, possibly pain and fistulae (Figure 56.2). Early findings on DPT and CT are sclerosis commonly affecting the alveolar margin, thickening of lamina dura and poor or non-healing extraction sockets. When established, osteonecrosis can be demonstrated on plain radiography and CT as mixed sclerosis and lysis, sequestra, bone fragmentation, pathological fracture, and soft-tissue swelling.

Osteonecrosis can be spontaneous – especially affecting a small area of the mylohyoid ridge.

• *Infections* (e.g. osteomyelitis).
• *Arteriovenous malformations.*
• *Central giant cell lesion* (grauloma) – consists of cellular fibrous tissue with multiple hemorrhagic foci, aggregations of multinucleated giant cells and occasionally trabeculae of woven bone. Most are asymptomatic but some are more aggressive, causing root resorption, pain or paresthesia, and cortical perforation (Figures 56.3a and b).
• *Fibro-osseous lesions* (Chapter 57).
• *Metabolic bone disorders* (e.g. osteomalacia, hyperparathyroidism).
• *Osteopetrosis.* A rare syndrome caused by osteoclast defects, this presents with excessive bone calcification, causing a marble-like radiopacity of the skeleton, and multiple fractures. Complications may also include jaw osteomyelitis, especially in the mandible (in 10%), anemia, hepatomegaly, and cranial nerve compression. Investigations include radiography and blood tests (low blood calcium, and often raised serum phosphatase). Management with vitamin D (calcitriol), gamma interferon, erythropoietin and corticosteroids may help.

Neoplastic disorders

• *Bone neoplasms* (Table 56.1).
• *Ewing sarcoma.* This is a rare malignant round-cell tumor mainly of young males, affecting bones and soft tissues, presenting as a radiolucent lesion with a lamellated or "onion skin" type of periosteal reaction. It is positive for CD99 (Cluster of Differentiation 99) marker. As many as 30% have metastasized by time of presentation. Chemotherapy gives a five-year survival for localized disease up to 80%, but only one-third of this if metastasized.

• *Langerhans cell histiocytoses* (LCH) or granulomatosis. Histiocytic disorders are divided into (1) dendritic cell histiocytosis, (2) erythrophagocytic macrophage disorders, and (3) malignant histiocytosis. LCH belongs to the first group and encompasses a number of diseases. These are rare disorders associated with a reactive increase in bone marrow-derived Langerhans cells (histiocytes – activated dendritic cells and macrophages) in the bone marrow (Figure 56.4), and sometimes in skin and other organs that can behave like a malignant disease. Major categories include:
— solitary, indolent and chronic, bone involvement – *eosinophilic granuloma*
— an intermediate form with multiple bone involvement, with or without skin involvement, characterized by multifocal, chronic involvement – classically the triad of diabetes insipidus, proptosis, and lytic bone lesions – *Hand-Schuller-Christian disease*
— acute fulminant, disseminated multiple organ involvement with bone and liver lesions – *Letterer-Siwe disease*
• *Leukemias.* Any of the five leukocyte types can be affected by malignant change – leukemia. The malignant leukocytes are dysfunctional (predisposing the patient to infections), and crowd other cells out of the bone marrow, so that frequently not enough normal blood cells are made. This leads to anemia because red cell production is impaired, and to excessive bleeding and bruising as platelets are impaired. Patients with leukemia present therefore with anemia, bruising and bleeding and liability to infections. Jaw involvement may include pain and swelling, or sensory disturbances. Imaging may confirm osteolytic lesions; expanded, coarse marrow spaces and trabeculae; alveolar bone destruction; loss of lamina dura and border of developmental dental crypts; and a periosteal reaction with an "onion skin" effect.
• *Myelodysplastic syndrome* (MDS) – diseases also characterized by abnormal bone marrow cell production and not enough normal blood cells are made, leading to anemia, infection, excessive bleeding and bruising. MDS are, in essence, pre-leukemia and leukemia may result.
• *Myeloproliferative disorders* (MPD) – diseases characterized by overproduction of precursor (immature form) marrow cells.
• *Plasma cell disorders.* These conditions (e.g. multiple myeloma) associated with overproduction of a B lymphocyte clone and its antibody, may affect the jaws. Radiographic findings include sharply defined radiolucencies usually of many bones, absence of marginal hyperostosis or opaque lining (Figure 56.5a and b).
• *Aplastic anemia* – associated with loss of cell precursors (usually erythrocytes) due to stem cell defects or injuries to the marrow environment.
• *Lymphomas.* Malignant diseases of lymphocytes, lymphomas and other cancers that spread into the bone marrow can affect cell production. Clinical presentation includes ill-defined radiolucency in bone.
• *Metastases.* The most frequent sites of primary neoplasms resulting in metastases are kidney, lung, breast, colon, prostate, and stomach. Metastases to the jaws are rare, usually to the posterior mandible, and typically manifest with pain and swelling, or sensory disturbances. Not uncommon are loosening of teeth, pathologic jaw fracture, or intraosseous lesions with lytic, ill-defined radiolucencies.

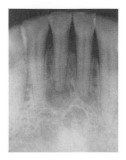

Figure 57.1a Periapical osseous dysplasia (early).

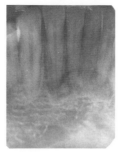

Figure 57.1b Periapical osseous dysplasia (mature).

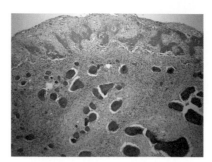

Figure 57.1c Focal osseous dysplasia histology.

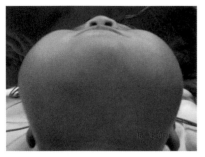

Figure 57.2a Cherubism.

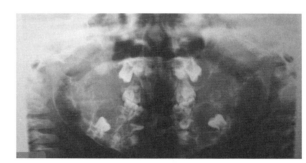

Figure 57.2b Cherubism.

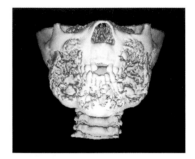

Figure 57.2c Cherubism.

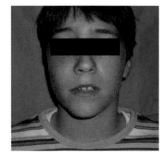

Figure 57.3a Fibrous dysplasia.

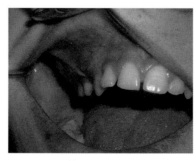

Figure 57.3b Fibrous dysplasia.

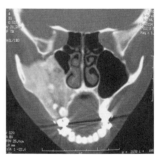

Figure 57.3c CT fibrous dysplasia.

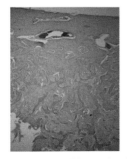

Figure 57.3d Fibrous dysplasia.

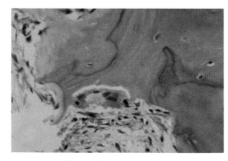

Figure 57.4 Paget disease.

Box 57.1 Fibro-osseous lesions.

Cemento-osseous dysplasia (osseous dysplasia)
Cherubism
Fibrous dysplasia
Hypercementosis
Ossifying fibroma
Paget disease of bone

Fibro-osseous lesions are a group of conditions characterized by replacement of normal bone by a proliferating fibrous stroma which forms varying amounts of woven bone spicules and cementum-like material (Box 57.1).

Osseous dysplasia, cemento-osseous dysplasia (COD), periapical cemental or cemento-osseous dysplasia (PCD)

Osseous dysplasia is a fibro-osseous lesion more common in females of African heritage during fourth and fifth decades, presenting with radiolucent and radiopaque lesions at the apices of vital teeth (periapical type), which may be isolated (focal) or multi-quadrant (florid). Lesions, which usually involve the mandibular anterior teeth, start as well-circumscribed radiolucent lesions and progressively become radiopaque centrally, although a thin radiolucent margin is usually visible (helpful in distinguishing from enostosis (idiopathic osteosclerosis)). The lesions are asymptomatic, usually incidental radiographic findings, and the related teeth are vital (Figures 57.1a–c). Florid COD is probably a widespread form, also occurring mainly in females of African heritage but usually affecting three or more quadrants. Bone expansion may occur, and the lesions may present with pain. Bone cysts may develop, and there is a liability to osteomyelitis. Sometimes COD occurs as isolated lesions unassociated with teeth (focal cemento-osseous dysplasia).

COD is self-limiting, so treatment is best limited to symptomatic relief of active infection and localized sequestration. In some cases of florid COD, surgical removal may be required.

Cherubism

The name for this comes from the appearance of angelic putti (chubby boys) in Renaissance art, misnamed by some as cherubs (Figures 57.2a–c). The mandible in particular is replaced with excessive fibrous tissue which usually resolves as the child matures. Rarely, it causes premature loss of primary teeth and uneruption of permanent teeth. Cherubism is an autosomal dominant condition involving SH3BP2 gene and has little in common with fibrous dysplasia.

Fibrous dysplasia

Fibrous dysplasia (FD) is a self-limiting fibro-osseous lesion caused by mutation in the gene encoding G protein (GNAS1). FD usually affects only one bone (monostotic, about 70%) but occasionally several (polyostotic). Maxillofacial FD may occur anywhere in the jaws but is essentially monostotic and typically affects the maxilla in young people, although it sometimes affects adjacent bones (*craniofacial fibrous dysplasia*), but rarely crosses the midline (Figures 57.3a–d). Bone enlarges in FD but the morphology is preserved, distinguishing FD from a neoplasm. CT can best assess the extent in the facial skeleton. FD lesions vary from radiolucent to radiopaque (often a "ground-glass appearance") with ill-defined margins – a feature helpful to distinguish it from other lesions. Histopathology shows woven bone directly forming from a fibrocellular background, fusing to adjacent cortical lamellar bone (Figure 57.3d).

Typically no treatment is needed. Bisphosphonates can help and surgery may be indicated if there is major deformity or pressure on nerves.

McCune-Albright's syndrome is FD bone lesions with skin pigmentation and endocrinopathy (precocious puberty in females and hyperthyroidism in males).

Hypercementosis

Hypercementosis is increased deposition of cementum on roots, caused by local trauma, inflammation, Paget disease, or it may occur idiopathically.

Ossifying fibroma (cemento-ossifying fibroma)

Ossifying fibroma is a usually benign, slow-growing, painless bone neoplasm, typically monostotic and seen in the third and fourth decades in the posterior mandible as a radiolucent, radiopaque, or mixed opacity which has a fibro-osseous microscopic appearance. Ossifying fibroma and focal COD are not easily differentiated histopathologically. Juvenile ossifying fibroma is an aggressive variant with a rapid growth pattern seen mainly in boys aged under 15 years.

Traditionally, the initial treatment has been surgical enucleation. More definitive resection has been reserved for recurrent disease.

Paget disease of bone

Paget disease of bone (PDB) is a progressive fibro-osseous disease affecting bone and cementum, characterized by disorganization of osteoclastogenesis (osteoclast formation), a process dependent on two cytokines – macrophage colony stimulating factor (M-CSF) and receptor activator of NF-kB ligand (RANKL), which induce gene expression changes, presumably by inducing transcription factors. The tumor necrosis factor (TNF) receptor superfamily activate nuclear factor κB (NF-κB), and RANK (receptor activator of NF-kappa B), which is involved in osteoclastogenesis.

Seen mainly in males over 55 years of age, there is a strong genetic component; 15%–20% have a first-degree relative with PDB. Genes involved include the sequestosome1 gene (SQSTM1).

In PDB, bone remodelling is disrupted, and an anarchic alternation of bone resorption and apposition results in mosaic-like "reversal lines", often associated with severe bone pain (Figure 57.4). In early lesions, bone destruction predominates (osteolytic stage) and there is bowing of the long bones, especially the tibia, pathological fractures, broadening/flattening of the chest and spinal deformity. The increased bone vascularity can lead to high output cardiac failure.

Later, as disease activity declines, bone apposition increases (osteosclerotic stage) and bones enlarge, with progressive thickening (between these phases is a mixed phase). PDB is typically polyostotic and may affect skull, skull base, sphenoid, orbital and frontal bones. The maxilla often enlarges, particularly in the molar region, with widening of the alveolar ridge. In early lesions, large irregular areas of relative radiolucency (osteoporosis circumscripta) are seen, but later there is increased radiopacity, with appearance of "cotton wool" pattern. Constriction of skull foraminae may cause cranial neuropathies. The dense bone and hypercementosis make tooth extraction difficult, and there is also a liability to hemorrhage and infection.

Diagnosis is supported by imaging, biochemistry and histopathology. Bone scintiscanning shows localized areas of high uptake. Plasma alkaline phosphatase and urine hydroxyproline levels increase with little or no changes in serum calcium or phosphate levels. Bisphosphonates are the treatment but calcitonin may also help.

58 Maxillary sinus conditions

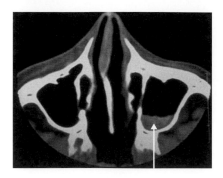

Figure 58.1a CT showing sinusitis.

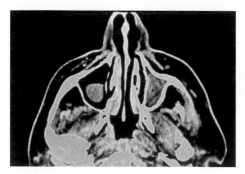

Figure 58.1b CT showing antral polp (right) and bacterial sinusitis (left).

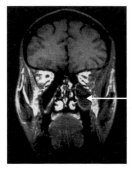

Figure 58.2 MRI showing antral aspergillosis.

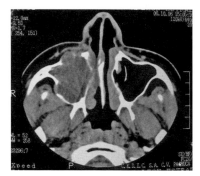

Figure 58.3 CT showing antral tumor.

Table 58.1 Classification of rhinosinusitis.

Rhinosinusitis type	Defined by duration
Acute	7 days to ≤ 4 weeks
Subacute	4–12 weeks
Recurrent acute	≥ 4 episodes of acute per year
Chronic	≥ 12 weeks
Acute exacerbation of chronic	Sudden worsening of chronic with later return to baseline

Report of the Rhinosinusitis Task Force Committee Meeting (1997). *Otolaryngology Head and Neck Surgery*, **117**, S1–68.

Box 58.1 Factors predisposing to sinusitis.

- allergic (vasomotor) rhinitis and nasal polyps
- viral upper respiratory tract infection (URTI)
  — diving or flying
  — nasal or antral foreign bodies
  — periapical infection of maxillary posterior teeth
  — oroantral fistula
  — prolonged endotracheal intubation

Table 58.2 Rhinosinusitis.

Location	Location of pain	Other features
Maxillary	Cheek and/or upper teeth	Tenderness over antrum
Frontal	Over frontal sinuses	Tenderness of sides of nose
Ethmoidal	Between eyes	Anosmia, eyelid swelling
Sphenoidal	Ear, neck, and at top or centre of head	—

Paranasal sinuses are air-filled cavities in the dense portions of the bones of the skull, lined with a ciliated mucosa, the mucus from which drains via openings (ostia) into the nose. The main sinuses are frontal, ethmoidal, sphenoidal and maxillary. Their main disorders are inflammatory and neoplastic. This chapter focuses on the maxillary sinus (antrum).

Rhinosinusitis (sinusitis)

Definition: Inflammation of the sinus mucosa (also involves the nose). Sinusitis most commonly affects the ethmoid sinuses, which then causes a secondary maxillary sinusitis. As a result of later development of the sinuses, sphenoid sinusitis is unusual in children under age five years and frontal sinusitis is unusual before age ten. Maxillary sinusitis is usually subdivided into acute and chronic sinusitis, but the classification is shown in Table 58.1.

Prevalence (approximate): Common (15–20% of the population at some point).

Age mainly affected: Any.

Gender mainly affected: M = F.

Etiopathogenesis: Cilia damage (e.g. tobacco smoke exposure), or impaired mucociliary clearance as when ostia are obstructed (e.g. allergic or infective rhinitis, foreign bodies, polyps). A change in sinus air pressure may cause pain (e.g. from ostia obstruction, increased mucus production, or air pressure changes such as flying or diving) (Box 58.1).

Bacteria are most commonly the cause, and the following are incriminated:

• In acute sinusitis, *Streptococcus pneumoniae*, *Haemophilus influenzae* and (in children) *Moraxella catarrhalis*, *Staphylococcus aureus* may be seen.

• In chronic sinusitis, also anaerobes, especially Porphyromonas (Bacteroides).

• In some circumstances, Gram-positive and Gram-negative organisms may be found – especially after prolonged endotracheal intubation, and in HIV/AIDS. In many immunocompromised persons, fungi (mucor, aspergillus or others) may be involved and, in cystic fibrosis, *Pseudomonas aeruginosa*, *Acinetobacter baumannii* and Enterobacteriaceae are often implicated.

Diagnostic features

History: Symptoms can include nasal drainage (rhinorrhea or post-nasal drip), nasal blockage, the sensation of swelling in nose or sinuses, ear symptoms, pain in teeth worse on biting or leaning over, halitosis, headache, fever, cough, malaise, etc. (Table 58.2). Symptoms are typically less severe in chronic sinusitis.

Clinical features

There may be nasal turbinate swelling, erythema and injection; mucus; sinus tenderness; allergic "shiners" (dark circles around eyes), pharyngeal erythema, otitis, etc.

Diagnosis is from the history, plus sinus tenderness and dullness on transillumination. Nasendoscopic-guided middle meatal cultures, or a sinus tap help sample infected material to determine the responsible micro-organisms.

CT is the standard of care in diagnosing chronic sinusitis (Figures 58.1a and b), but differentiating from upper respiratory tract infection is difficult. Antral radiopacities in children under age six years can be difficult to evaluate since they are seen in up to 50%. In adults, a sinus radiopacity may be due to mucosal thickening, but a fluid level is highly suggestive. MRI may be helpful.

In patients with recurrent or recalcitrant sinusitis, fungal infections (Figure 58.2), cystic fibrosis and immunodeficiencies may need to be excluded.

Management

Acute sinusitis resolves spontaneously in about 50%, but analgesics are often indicated and other therapies may be required, especially if symptoms persist or there is purulent discharge. Intranasal steroids can be helpful, although studies have not been conclusive. Antihistamines are used for significant allergic symptoms. Oral decongestants help, but should be used for 3–7 days only, as longer use may cause rebound and rhinitis medicamentosa. Guaifenesin helps clearance of secretions. Buffered saline lavage may help in clearing secretions. Hot steam may help.

Antibiotics are required for at least two weeks in acute sinusitis – amoxicillin (or ampicillin or co-amoxiclav), or a tetracycline such as doxycycline, or clindamycin. Chronic sinusitis responds best to drainage by functional endoscopic sinus surgery (FESS), plus antimicrobials (metronidazole with amoxicillin, clindamycin or a cephalosporin) for at least three weeks. Open procedures including the classical Caldwell-Luc operation are generally outmoded.

Neoplasms

Definition: Usually squamous carcinoma.

Prevalence (approximate): Rare.

Age mainly affected: Older people.

Gender mainly affected: M > F.

Etiopathogenesis: Exposure to wood dust, nickel, chromium, polycyclic hydrocarbons, aflatoxin and thorotrast (thorium dioxide used in paints for watch dials) have been implicated.

Diagnostic features

These tumors can remain undetected until late. When they infiltrate branches of the trigeminal nerve they cause maxillary pain. As the tumor expands the effects of expansion and infiltration of adjacent tissues become apparent as intraoral alveolar swelling, ulceration of the palate or buccal sulcus; swelling of the cheek; unilateral nasal obstruction often associated with a blood-stained discharge; obstruction of the nasolacrimal duct with epiphora; hypo- or anesthesia of the cheek; proptosis and ophthalmoplegia consequent on invasion of the orbit and trismus from infiltration of the muscles of mastication.

Diagnosis is supported by endoscopy, radiography (Figure 58.3), magnetic resonance imaging, and biopsy.

Management

Combinations of surgery (maxillectomy) and radiochemotherapy are usually required.

Prognosis is poor, with a < 30% five-year survival, not least because presentation is often late.

59 Oral malodor

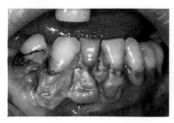

Figure 59.1 Chronic periodontitis and massive calculus deposits.

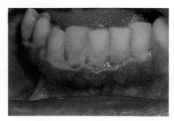

Figure 59.2 Acute necrotizing ulcerative gingivitis is particularly odiferous.

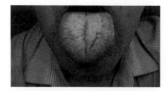

Figure 59.4a Tongue coating.

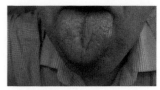

Figure 59.4b Tongue coating after scraping and brushing.

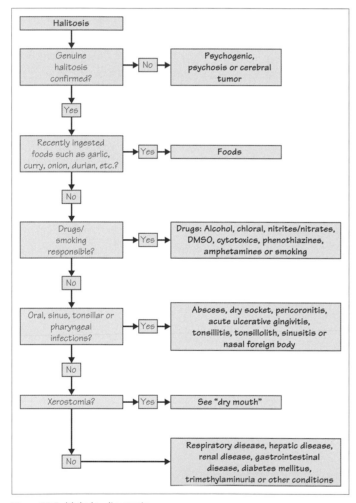

Figure 59.3 Malodor diagnosis.

Flowchart:

Halitosis

Genuine halitosis confirmed? — No → Psychogenic, psychosis or cerebral tumor

Yes ↓

Recently ingested foods such as garlic, curry, onion, durian, etc.? — Yes → Foods

No ↓

Drugs/smoking responsible? — Yes → Drugs: Alcohol, chloral, nitrites/nitrates, DMSO, cytotoxics, phenothiazines, amphetamines or smoking

No ↓

Oral, sinus, tonsillar or pharyngeal infections? — Yes → Abscess, dry socket, pericoronitis, acute ulcerative gingivitis, tonsillitis, tonsillolith, sinusitis or nasal foreign body

No ↓

Xerostomia? — Yes → See "dry mouth"

No ↓

Respiratory disease, hepatic disease, renal disease, gastrointestinal disease, diabetes mellitus, trimethylaminuria or other conditions

---

Box 59.1 Main oral causes of malodor.

Plaque-related gingival and periodontal disease
Ulceration
Hyposalivation
Tongue coating
Dental appliances
Dental infections
Bone infections

Box 59.2 Main extraoral causes of malodor.

Respiratory system
Gastrointestinal system
Metabolic disorders
Drugs
Psychogenic causes

Definition: Oral malodor or halitosis (Latin halitus = breath) describes any disagreeable breath odor. Descriptive terms are shown in Table 59.1.

Prevalence (approximate): Up to 30% of population.

Age mainly affected: Adults.

Gender mainly affected: M > F.

Etiopathogenesis: Common on awakening (morning breath), in starvation, and with various foods and habits but is then transient and rarely significant.

Malodor originates from the mouth, mainly from poor oral hygiene (Figure 59.1), ulcers or infections (Figure 59.2), in about 85% of patients affected (Box 59.1).

Halitosis arises from micro-organism activity; no single specific bacterial infection has invariably been associated, but anaerobes, *Prevotella* species, *Solobacterium moorei* on the tongue and other potentially novel phylotypes have been implicated. The odiferous products that cause halitosis appear to be produced mainly in the mouth, usually from microbial interactions with specific substrates biotransforming them into volatile sulphur compounds; VSCs (such as hydrogen sulphide, methylmercaptan), indoles such as tryptamine and skatole, and polyamines (putrescine and cadaverine). Short chain fatty acids (e.g. valerate, propionate and butyrate) may also arise.

Halitosis is much less frequently associated with extraoral causes (Box 59.2).

Diagnostic features

The first step is to decide whether malodor is present, usually by the organoleptic assessment of exhaled air – the clinician sniffs air exhaled from the mouth and nose. Malodor detectable from the nose alone (the patient breathes with the mouth closed) is likely to originate from nose, sinuses, tonsils, respiratory or gastrointestinal tracts. More objective measurements of malodor (gas chromatography; sulphide monitoring with a halimeter) are expensive and time-consuming. If no malodor is found at the initial examination, the assessment should be repeated on two different days.

Thereafter, if malodor is still not detectable, the patient is considered to have pseudo-halitosis. If malodor is present, the cause should be established (Figure 59.3) (Table 59.2).

Management

Smoking, drugs, and foods that might be responsible for odor should be avoided. Regular meals are important. In most patients, treatment is directed towards reducing the accumulation of food debris and malodor-producing oral bacteria, achieved by treating oral/dental diseases, reducing the tongue coating by brushing/scraping (Figures 59.4a and b), improving oral hygiene – tooth cleaning (brushing and interdental flossing) and use of antimicrobial toothpastes and/or mouthwashes (chlorhexidine gluconate, ceptylpyridinium chloride, zinc or triclosan, may be beneficial). Chewing gum, parsley, mint, cloves or fennel seeds and the use of proprietary "fresh breath" preparations may help temporarily mask the unfavourable odor. A combination of treatments typically helps.

In recalcitrant cases, the specialist empirically may use a course of metronidazole in an effort to eliminate unidentified anaerobic infections. Oral malodor due to extraoral causes is managed through treatment of the underlying cause (Table 59.2). Medical help may be required to manage patients with a systemic background to their complaint.

Prognosis

No evidence on oral malodor prognosis has been published to date.

Table 59.1 Terminology related to oral malodor.

Terms used	Definition	
Halitosis	Any disagreeable breath malodor	
Genuine halitosis	Breath malodor objectively verified	
	Physiologic (transient) breath malodor, e.g. morning breath	Pathologic breath malodor
Pseudo-halitosis	No objective evidence of breath malodor	
Halitophobia	Patient persists in believing they have breath malodor despite firm evidence for absence of objective halitosis	

Table 59.2 Diagnostic sequence for malodor.

Medical speciality	More common diseases and predisposing conditions	Diagnostic techniques
Dentistry	Abscesses Food impaction Gingivitis Neoplasms Periodontitis Poor oral hygiene Tongue coating Ulcers	Physical examination Plaque and gingival bleeding indices Periodontal probing Periapical radiography Breath odiferous compounds quantification (1)
Otorhinolaryngology/pneumology	*Upper respiratory tract* Sinusitis Antral malignancy Cleft palate Foreign bodies in the nose Nasal malignancy Tonsilloliths Tonsillitis Pharyngeal malignancy *Lower respiratory tract* Lung infections Bronchitis Bronchiectasis Lung malignant disease	Physical examination Sinus radiography nasendoscopy Microbiological study Computed tomography (1) Magnetic resonance imaging (1) Nasal smears (1) Thorax radiography Bronchoscopy (1)
Digestive system	Zenker diverticulum Extrinsic duodenal obstructions Pyloric stenosis Gastric fistula *Helicobacter pylori* Hepatic cirrhosis (foetor hepaticus) Esophageal diverticulum Gastro esophageal reflux disease Malignancy	Physical examination Plain abdomen radiography Barium studies ^{13}c-urea breath test Endoscopy (1) Transaminase levels Viral hepatitis serology Liver echography
Endocrinology	Cystinosis Diabetes (acetone-like smell in uncontrolled diabetes) Hypermethioninemia Trimethylaminuria (fish odor syndrome)	Physical examination Glucose tolerance test Glycemia Ketonic compounds determination Trimethylamine levels in urine (1) Methioninemia determination (1)
Nephrology	Renal insufficiency (final stage) Uremic breath in renal failure	Physical examination Uremia and nitrogenous compound levels Breath dimethyl- and trimethyl-amine levels determination (1)
Neuropsychiatry	Olfactory illusion syndrome (delusionary halitosis) Monosymptomatic hypochondriac psychosis Temporal lobe epilepsy Cyclic phantosmia Schizophrenia	Physical examination Specific neurologic evaluation Specific psychiatric evaluation

(1) complementary diagnostic techniques of second choice.

60 Human immunodeficiency virus (HIV) infection and AIDS

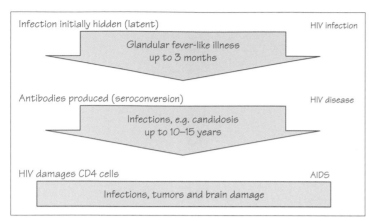

Infection initially hidden (latent)	HIV infection
Glandular fever-like illness up to 3 months	
Antibodies produced (seroconversion)	HIV disease
Infections, e.g. candidosis up to 10–15 years	
HIV damages CD4 cells	AIDS
Infections, tumors and brain damage	

Figure 60.1 HIV infection progression.

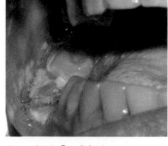

Figure 60.2 Candidosis.

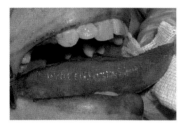

Figure 60.3 Hairy leukoplakia.

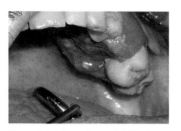

Figure 60.4 Lymphoma in HIV disease.

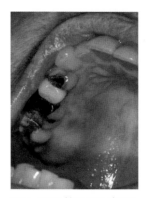

Figure 60.5 Herpetic ulcers.

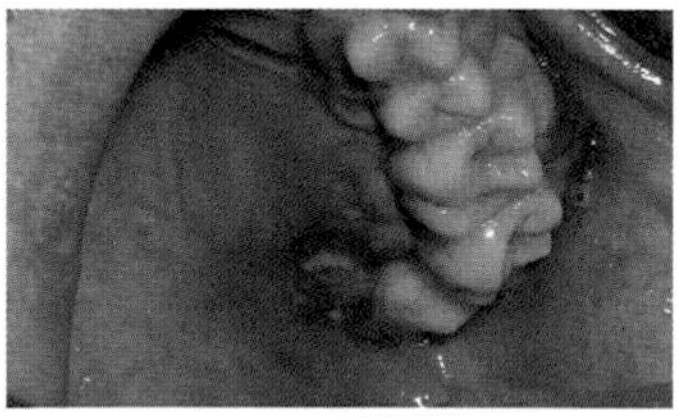

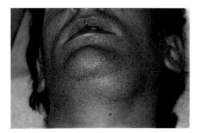

Figure 60.6a Kaposi sarcoma.

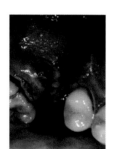

Figure 60.6b Kaposi sarcoma.

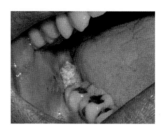

Figure 60.7 Human papillomavirus infection.

Figure 60.8 Tuberculosis sialadenitis.

Definitions: A retrovirus infection leading to severe CD4 T lymphocyte defects and opportunistic infections (HIV disease). There are two main viruses: HIV-1 is by far the most common but HIV-2 has spread mainly from West Africa. Acquired Immune Deficiency Syndrome (AIDS) is the term used when the CD4 count falls < 200 cells/ul (Centers for Disease Control and Prevention, USA). The World Health Organization (WHO), however, included in the AIDS case definition the following criteria:

• 10% body weight loss or cachexia, with diarrhea or fever, or both, intermittent or constant for at least one month, not known to be due to a condition unrelated to HIV infection
• cryptococcal meningitis
• tuberculosis, pulmonary or extra-pulmonary
• Kaposi sarcoma
• neurological impairment sufficient to prevent independent daily activities, not known to be due to a condition unrelated to HIV infection
• candidosis (esophageal)
• pneumonia, clinically diagnosed, life-threatening or recurrent, with or without etiological confirmation
• cervical cancer (invasive)

Prevalence (approximate): In 2007, 33.2 million people were estimated to be living with HIV, 2.5 million people became newly infected and 2.1 million people died of AIDS; up to 50% of populations in southern Africa are infected.

Age mainly affected: Adults or children.

Gender mainly affected: F = M worldwide; also common in men who have sex with men (MSM).

Etiopathogenesis: HIV infects cells with CD4 receptors (T-helper lymphocytes and brain glial cells), which become dysfunctional and die, producing progressive immune deficiency and dementia (Figure 60.1).

Defenses become impaired, especially against fungi, viruses, mycobacteria and parasites. Clinical disease (HIV disease) manifests after a long latency, with tumors, infections and other features.

HIV is present in tissues and body fluids (including blood and saliva) of HIV-infected persons, constituting an infective risk.

Diagnostic features
History
Oral. Acute HIV infection can cause fever, malaise, lymphadenopathy, and myalgia (mimicking glandular fever). HIV infection is then asymptomatic, often for years, until symptomatic (HIV disease) and then AIDS eventually appears, with serious infections and neoplasms.

Extraoral: Weight loss ("slim disease") and diarrhea.

Clinical features
Oral: Candidosis (Figure 60.2) and hairy leukoplakia (Figure 60.3) are most common, but other lesions may also be seen (Table 60.1).

Mouth ulcers in HIV/AIDS may be due to aphthous-like ulcers; infections (mainly herpesviruses or necrotizing gingivitis/periodontitis, but occasionally mycobacteria, syphilis, Rochalimaea, Histoplasma, Cryptococcus, Leishmania) or malignant disease (mainly Kaposi sarcoma or non-Hodgkin lymphoma).

Extraoral: infections and neoplasms are seen (Table 60.2).

Differential diagnosis: Other immune defects, especially leukemias.

Investigations
HIV serotesting is mandatory, after counseling. Seroconversion occurs, usually within 30–50 days of infection. The enzyme-linked immunosorbent assay (ELISA) for HIV p24 antibodies is the main test, but must be repeated and may need to be confirmed by Western blot. False test reactions are rare. HIV RNA is a measure of the viral load (HIV copy numbers of virus per unit of blood).

Blood tests: CD4 count < 500/ul is indicative of immunosuppression. CD4+ lymphocyte counts of < 200 are indicators of imminent opportunistic infection and signals to commence antimicrobial chemoprophylaxis.

Management
Medical: Antiretroviral therapy (ART), which can prolong life, includes:
• *Nucleoside analogue reverse transcriptase inhibitors (NARTI)*:
  — zidovudine (AZT)
  — didanosine (DDI)
  — zalcitabine (DDC)
  — lamivudine (3TC)
• *Non-nucleoside analogue reverse transcriptase inhibitors*:
  — nevirapine
• *Protease inhibitors*:
  — saquinavir
  — ritonavir
  — indinavir
• *Integrase inhibitors*:
  — raltegravir
• *Fusion inhibitors*:
  — enfuvirtide
  — maraviroc

Combination ART (CART) has increased life expectancy. Protease inhibitors (PIs) are used together with reverse transcriptase inhibitors as highly active ART (HAART), which has reduced infections and extended life. Serious conditions such as Kaposi sarcoma resolve spontaneously but drug effects cause more morbidity than AIDS itself. However, there may be a temporary paradoxical immunoinflammatory reaction (termed immune reconstitution inflammatory syndrome (IRIS)) brought about by improved immune status following HAART, and some infections (e.g. herpes zoster and HPV-induced warts) have increased. Oral lesions in IRIS include major salivary gland swelling, candidosis, herpes labialis, necrotizing periodontitis, xerostomia, hairy leukoplakia, and oral ulceration.

Prognosis
Premature death is inevitable. Vaccines against HIV are in their infancy.

Table 60.1 Orofacial lesions in HIV disease.

Etiological agent		Main examples	Manifestations
Infection	**Viral**	Epstein-Barr virus	Ulcers, lymphoma (Figure 60.4), hairy leukoplakia (Figure 60.3)
		Herpes simplex	Ulcers (Figure 60.5)
		Herpes varicella zoster	Ulcers, pain
		Kaposi sarcoma associated herpesvirus	Kaposi sarcoma (Figures 60.6a and b)
		Human papillomaviruses	Papillomas or warts (Figure 60.7)
	Fungal	Aspergillus	
		Candida (Figure 60.2)	White or red lesions, ulcers
		Histoplasma capsulatum	Lump
	Bacterial	*Mycobacterium tuberculosis*	Ulcers, lumps, lymphadenopathy
		Non-tuberculous mycobacteria	Ulcers, lump, lymphadenopathy
		Periodontal flora	Necrotizing gingivitis and periodontitis
	Protozoal	Leishmania	Ulcers, lump
Autoimmune		Aphthous-like ulcers	
		Salivary gland swelling (Figure 60.8), e.g. from diffuse infiltrative lymphocytosis syndrome (DILS)*, or multiple lymphoepithelial cysts	
		Xerostomia	
Other		Erythema multiforme	
		Exfoliative cheilitis	
		Facial palsy	
		Hyperpigmentation	
		Taste disturbance	
		Trigeminal neuralgia	

* Involves salivary glands, lungs, kidneys and gastrointestinal tract.

Table 60.2 Extraoral lesions in HIV disease.

Etiological agent		Main examples	Manifestations
Infection	**Viral**	Cytomegalovirus	Eyes, disseminated
		Epstein-Barr virus	Lymphoma
		Herpes simplex	Perianal, disseminated
		Herpes varicella zoster	Zoster
		Kaposi sarcoma associated herpesvirus	Kaposi sarcoma
		Human papillomavirus	Papillomas or warts
	Fungal	Aspergillus	
		Candida	Candidosis (esophagus, bronchi or lung)
		Histoplasma capsulatum	Disseminated
		Coccidioidomycosis	
		Cryptococcosis	Disseminated
		Pneumocystis carinii (jirovecii)	Brain, disseminated pneumonia
	Bacterial	Cryptosporidiosis	Gastrointestinal
		Isosporiasis	
		Mycobacterium tuberculosis	Respiratory and disseminated
		Non-tuberculous mycobacteria	Respiratory and disseminated
	Protozoal	Leishmania	Skin
		Toxoplasmosis	Brain
Autoimmune		Purpura	
Other		Diarrhea	
		Fatigue	
		Fever	
		Lymphadenopathy	
		Malaise	
		Splenomegaly	
		Thrombocytopenia	
		Wasting	
		Weight loss	

Index

Page numbers in **bold** represent tables, those in *italics* represent figures.